Praise for *Year of No Sugar*

"As an outspoken advocate of healthy eating, I found Schaub's book to shine a much-needed spotlight on an aspect of American culture that is making us sick, fat, and unhappy, and it does so with wit and warmth."

—Suvir Saran, author of *Indian Home Cooking*

"The surface charm of *Year of No Sugar*—breezy wit, blithe anecdote, and effortless evocation of people and the stuff they put in their mouths—cannot conceal Schaub's deeper purpose: a takedown of sugar, its disarming myths, its dangerous presence in nearly everything we eat, and its cynical marketing. Delicious and compelling, her book is just about the best sugar substitute I've ever encountered."

—Pulitzer Prize–winning author Ron Powers

"Eve O. Schaub's *Year of No Sugar* has the potential to alter your deeply rooted convictions regarding the innocent pleasure of sugar."

—Betsy Shaw, BabyCenter.com blogger
and former Olympic snowboarder

YEAR OF NO SUGAR

A Memoir

EVE O. SCHAUB

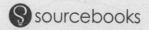

Published by Sourcebooks, Inc.
P.O. Box 4410, Naperville, Illinois 60567-4410
(630) 961-3900
Fax: (630) 961-2168
www.sourcebooks.com

Library of Congress Cataloging-in-Publication data is on file with the publisher.

Printed and bound in the United States of America.
WOZ 10 9 8 7 6 5 4 3 2 1

To Steve, Greta, and Ilsa,
without whom nothing is sweet

"It is remarkable how easily and insensibly we fall into a particular route, and make a beaten track for ourselves."

—Henry David Thoreau, *Walden*

CONTENTS

FOREWORD

Ten years ago my wife, Lizzie, did a very annoying thing. Without any consultation and without seeking any of the proper approvals from management, she decided to turn our fifth child into twins. One day, she was pregnant with baby #5, and the next, our world was turned upside down. We were about to add twin babies to our other four children (all under the age of nine at the time).

I was ninety pounds overweight and barely coping with the four we had, let alone chucking twins in. I was apathetic, moody (or so people tell me), and had just enough energy to stay at work until after the kids were in bed. Twin babies were not going to be fun. Unfortunately, pregnancy is one of those nonnegotiable forces of nature. There would be no extensions; come September 2003, we would be the parents of six children. I decided I needed to do something about my health, and in particular, I needed to stop being so fat.

I hadn't woken up one morning and discovered ninety extra pounds hanging off my waist. It had been a slow and inevitable accumulation. I had been working on that spare tire for the better part of three decades. Every now and then I would decide that enough was enough. I'd see a cabbage soup diet on TV or read about [insert name of very famous and inspiring person here] going on this or that diet. So I'd break out the cabbage or the bananas or delete the carbs or <gasp> go to the gym. And they would all work. I'd drop a pound or two a week for exactly as long as my willpower would hold out (usually about two weeks—what can I say? I'm weak). Then I would stop, and the weight would come back, usually with interest.

But this time I was determined. I decided I needed to understand how my body worked. I needed to understand why humans (and the animals they feed) were the only species on the planet that required willpower to control their weight. I needed to know why there were no tigers joining Weight Watchers and why there were no gyms for monkeys.

I was (and am) a lawyer, so I assumed it was just my lack of acquaintance with biochemistry that was ensuring I misapplied my various weight-loss techniques. I decided I needed to read deeply on the subject and not stop until I had the answer. Fortunately, I am related to approximately half the medical profession, so I had plenty of people telling me where to start (and stop) reading.

Once I got my head around the mind-bendingly arcane language, I discovered that scientists knew an awful lot about why I was fat. They knew that sugar was the cause. They knew that fat was the least worrying aspect of consuming sugar. They knew it caused type II diabetes and fatty liver disease and hypertension and chronic kidney disease and even Alzheimer's. And worst of all, they knew it was highly addictive and (because of this) being added liberally to the food supply. It didn't matter whether the sugar was made from corn (HFCS) or grass (cane sugar) or beets (the sugar they sell in Europe); it all contained the molecule responsible for the damage—fructose.

I didn't know any of this because it seemed that, rather like the tobacco companies, the folks making money out of pumping our food full of fructose were working very hard to ensure we looked at everything other than sugar. They told us it was our fault we were fat. We were lard buckets because we couldn't exercise self-control or because we didn't have the willpower to go to the gym every day. We had a character defect, and under no circumstances was it anything to do with the sugar.

I decided all I needed to do, if the science was right, was stop eating sugar. So I did. And magic happened. After a few weeks of ugliness involving intense cravings, some headaches, and staying well away from the soda fridge at the supermarket, I was suddenly not drawn to sugar. People would offer me chocolate, and I would say no without a cringe of regret. Willpower no longer seemed necessary. I was applying just one rule: if it's sweet, don't eat. But other than that, I ate whatever I wanted. And the truly miraculous thing was that I was losing weight. Every week the scales would drop another couple of pounds, but I was doing all the wrong things. I wasn't exercising, I was eating as much fatty food as I wanted, and I was even eating cheese! Magic.

A year or so later, I was ninety pounds lighter. I can't tell you exactly how long it took or exactly what the process was. I can't tell you precisely when Lizzie decided to join in my little sugar-free party or when she decided to bring the kids along. I can't tell you any of these things because I wasn't writing it down. I wasn't a blogger (was anyone in 2003?)

and I wasn't a writer. I was a lawyer with a day job who was obsessing about medical studies at night, and I certainly didn't have time to record what I was doing (as if anyone would be interested anyway).

Five years later, I did write a book about the science that had spurred me to action (*Sweet Poison*, Penguin Australia 2008), but I did that simply because it was clear that the science that I had read was not making it past the food industry PR filters, and something needed to be done about it. A book was the only medium I could think of that could not be influenced by the needs of advertisers or sponsors. But *Sweet Poison* is not a diary. It is a translation of the science. It doesn't have the detail which every prospective sugar quitter craves. It can't tell you if it's normal for your kids to despair at their parents' insane obsession with food. It can't tell you how to deal with a school system pumping your neighbors' kids full of sugar as a reward. It can't tell you how to be sugar free in a society obsessed with sugar. But this book can—and does.

I first discovered Eve's online diary of her sugar-free adventures about a month into her journey. By then, I was terribly famous in Australia (no, really, I was), and the sugar quitting concept was becoming quite mainstream there. So I was used to discovering blogs written by people who were quitting sugar. But Eve's blog was different. The detail was exquisite, and I loved her down-to-earth, we-are-just-plain-doing-this approach. I loved reading about the adventures of her family, the roadblocks they encountered, and the sheer daily difficulty of overcoming a national obsession. It reminded me of so many of the situations Lizzie and I had lived through but that I had never written down. It was the diary I wish I had kept.

Now, that blog has become this superb book. Background details have been filled in. Even more color and nuance has worked its way into the story, and Eve has shown herself to be a spectacularly good writer when she takes off the shackles of fitting it all into a weekly blog post. I am certain you will enjoy Eve's story but, even more importantly, I am certain it will provide all the motivation you need to take you and your family down the sugar-free road to a better (and longer) life. Enjoy!

—David Gillespie, author of *Sweet Poison*,
The Sweet Poison Quit Plan, *Big Fat Lies*,
and the website howmuchsugar.com

CHAPTER 1

I LOVE SUGAR

Sugar and me? We go way back.

I love sugar. LOOOOVVVVVE it. I love everything about it: how it makes little occasions special and special occasions fabulous. How it performs hot, bubbling magic on sour fruits, like rhubarb and gooseberries, to make the most succulent, mind-blowing pies and jams. How it crunches with perfect granulation in the best cookies and how a single cube of it adds fairy-tale perfection to a real Italian cappuccino.

And don't even get me *started* on chocolate.

I've known about the power of sugar for a long time. When I was in seventh grade, we were given an English-class assignment: create a "how-to" presentation on a subject of our choosing. Although I was awkward, painfully shy, and *terrified* to stand before the class, I still knew exactly what I wanted to do: a demonstration of different methods of cake decorating using a standard two-layer I had baked as a prop. Easy peasy.

The day of our presentations arrived, and I was petrified but excited—after all, I thought, how could I go wrong with a topic like *cake*? Then it came to be my turn and I, decked out in my best Esprit sweatshirt and ribbon barrettes, proceeded to inform the class how they could make their cakes more beautiful and interesting, which I'm sure had my preadolescent classmates simply *riveted*. This was *1982*, mind you, before Martha Stewart did for homemaking what Edward Cullen did for being alarmingly pale. Making cakes and cookies wasn't even remotely cool; it was what grannies did when they weren't crocheting throw blankets in shades of mustard and avocado.

Nonetheless, everything seemed to be going along fairly well until I got to the part about making designs in the frosting using the tines of a fork. After chocolate shavings and shaking powdered sugar through a doily, this was pretty much my Big Finish. It was then that I realized—with horror—that I had *Forgotten. The. Fork.*

Oh.

This was one in a series of moments in seventh grade when I fervently wished I had a shell in which to curl up and disappear, but lacking that, I instead turned a lovely shade of beet and attempted to *mime* the fork part. Worse public speaking debacles have happened, I imagine, but you couldn't have convinced me of that then.

However, despite the Fork Faux Pas and my appalling lack of public speaking skills, all was not lost. My English teacher *liked* the speech, but she *loved* the cake. I have a distinct memory of her pink, round face beaming as we all dug into our slices.[1] I received what was in all likelihood a wholly

---

[1] Wait, what did we eat our slices with? 'Cause that was the crux of the story—I had no fork, right? Honestly, I have no idea. Maybe we used spoons? Our fingers? Chopsticks?

undeserved A. That was proof enough for me in the power of sweet.

As far back as I can remember, I've *always* loved to bake. Once, when I was perhaps seven or eight years old, I created a carefully hand-lettered menu and invited everyone in the family to my "restaurant." Forensic analysis of that menu now reveals that I let Mom worry about the incidental entree of steak and baked potato (yeah, whatever), while I focused on what was *really* important: *apple cobbler for dessert.* The menu even featured a fanciful illustration of the *pièce de résistance* on the cover. As far as *I* was concerned, I had made dinner.

Like most kids, I knew dessert was something special, something magical. Every once in a while, my mother would handily transform a pile of fruit into a pie, handing us down the pastry scraps, which my brother and I would roll into little balls and eat raw while we climbed trees in the backyard. I pined for an Easy-Bake Oven in which to make my very own magical concoctions, but sadly, Santa ignored my culinary aspirations (also, my request for a Barbie Styling Head and Wonder Woman Underoos). So I pestered my mom to let me use the *real* oven until she finally relented.

I made box cakes from the time I could reach the kitchen counter. I remember my shock the first time flour exploded high into the air because I turned the mixer on too high, too fast; my cavernous disappointment the first time I tried to make a recipe without a key ingredient (baking powder, perhaps? I mean, how important could that half a teaspoon *really* be?), and it came out like warmed-over mud.

Still, I would bake at the drop of a hat—for our family, for the neighbor, for the neighbor's dog, for anyone. Everyone always loved it when I baked, with the possible exception of Mom, who patiently cleaned up after me. After all, who doesn't like dessert? Dessert to me was, and is, an ultimate expression of love—it is beyond a meal; it is beyond sustenance. It is something extra, something special that is made because someone simply wanted you to have it... More than being fed, they wanted you to be *happy*. I made the connection at an early age that sugar *is* the food equivalent of love.

I also learned that the withholding of sugar is a mighty punishment. Once, when we had a rather unobservant babysitter, I had the idea to bring a pocketful of the sparkly doodads from Mom's jewelry box to the playground and use them to decorate my sandbox creations. Of course, once I ran off distractedly to play elsewhere, the jewelry disappeared, and suddenly I found myself in big, *huge*, **ENORMOUS** trouble.

Abject, tear-stained, I waited like an inmate for my sentence. At last it came down from the powers that be: no dessert. For a *month*.

This may not sound like much to you, but believe me, it was the most effective punishment they could possibly have dreamed up. I was open-mouth *horrified*. A *month*? That was like, *forever*. I might *expire* first. Couldn't they just cane me instead?

But watching my family eat the occasional Entenmann's slice of yellow-sheet-cake-with-the-frosting-that-comes-right-off-in-one-piece wasn't the worst part. The *worst* part was that this, *this* was the month of a very special event: the Indian Princess Make-Your-Own-Sundae Party.

Oh. My. God.

I had never been to a Make-Your-Own-Ice-Cream-Sundae Party, but at that time, it only sounded to me like the Best Thing in the Whole World. I was more than horrified;

I was in shock. "Indian Princesses" was a YMCA-sponsored activity (and, obviously, a pre-politically correct era one at that). It was not unlike Brownies or Girl Scouts in that there were lots of craft projects and we marched together in local parades. But the main idea of Indian Princesses was that it was a father-daughter bonding activity, so I knew it was Dad who would be taking me. Would he break down? I wondered. Wouldn't he cave just a little at the sight of so much potential happiness just beyond his adorable little Indian Princess's reach?

The answer to that, actually, was no. Although my dad is known to be a bit of a softy, I'm guessing my mother prepped him in advance: no dessert means…No. Dessert. End of story. I sat and watched all my friends *and* their dads pile bowls high with what seemed to me at the time to be just about the most delicious combination of ingredients I had ever witnessed—not *just* ice cream and sprinkles, but M&M's, hot fudge and butterscotch, even *whipped cream from a can*! ARRRGGH!!!!!!! I was in Hell.

Let me just tell you, I *never* touched my mother's things *again*. Ever.

Since then, a lot of time has passed; over my teenage, college, and early adult years, I continued to bake and even became interested in actual meal cooking as well. No one I knew in college seemed quite as interested in these things as I was. Most everyone I knew was content to be spoon-fed whatever was trucked in to the myriad dining halls we had on campus. I insisted on going off the meal plan and doing my own food experimenting in the dorm mini-kitchen across the hall. While my floor-mates were discovering Jell-O shots or arguing over their Dungeons and Dragons powers,

I was making hummus in my room, buying bulk quinoa at the co-op downtown, and trying to figure out how to devein shrimp on top of my bedspread. When the apple pie I had baked from scratch for a friend's birthday was stolen from the communal fridge, I was beside myself. Stolen!! Pie tin and all—*gone*! Pinching money I could almost understand, but food? *Dessert*? A *birthday* dessert!?! Did these barbarians have no *humanity*?

Of course they didn't. We were talking about young adults whose idea of gourmet cuisine was mozzarella sticks from the Hot Truck. From an early age, I was long out of step with my peers when it came to my passion for food.

At the same time, I've been extremely lucky in life never to be in real need of losing weight, so food fads have come and gone without my feeling the need to pay much mind. The Low-Carb Diet, the Low-Fat Diet, the Atkins Diet, the South Beach Diet, the Blood Type Diet, the Eat All the Liver and Pistachios You Want Diet…I ignored them all. The only one that grabbed my attention in the late nineties was the popular Sugar Busters diet, which dictated that followers give up refined sugar and white flour.

"Why not just give up eating!?!" I would scoff to myself whenever an acquaintance would profess to have lost "a ton" of weight on Sugar Busters. I was annoyed. I was *offended* at the suggestion that cakes and pies—*my* cakes, *my* pies— made from scratch, with *love*, could be harmful. Harmful! "This is all going too far. What, are we never supposed to have *fun* anymore?"

Seriously. What harm could possibly be done by enjoying *dessert*?

CHAPTER 2

OUT OF THE OPIUM DEN

"How did this thing, this spice, sugar, become a staple? How did something that ought to be like saffron, a rare thing to add, become the thing we build on? How did a whole way of cooking creep up from sweetness?"

—White House Pastry Chef Bill Yosses[2]

The morning I watched the YouTube video "Sugar: The Bitter Truth," my brain caught fire.

"Hey, Eve, come watch this! You're gonna want to see this!"

My husband was calling to me from upstairs. There was a video posted on Facebook with some doctor droning on about sugar and health. *Well, how compelling can this be?* I thought. But Steve had watched several minutes of it and was transfixed.

So we watched it together for about twenty minutes. My husband left to go to work while I stayed and watched it to the end, ninety minutes total. Ninety minutes, as it turned

---

[2]Adam Gopnik, "Sweet Revolution," *The New Yorker*, January 3, 2011, 51.

out, that would change my life, and the life of our family, forever.

Dr. Robert Lustig is an unassuming-looking fellow with a medium build, gray hair, and a laser-like focus. He's good with PowerPoint and is comfortable throwing about phrases like "multivariate linear regression analysis." As "Sugar: The Bitter Truth" opens, he stands at a lectern in an anonymous-looking hall, looking every bit like that professor whose chemistry lectures put you to sleep every time. You'd never suspect that a ninety-minute educational lecture from this man could generate some three and a half million hits, but that's just what happened.

"I'm going to tell you, tonight, a story," Lustig begins. "By the end of the story, I hope I will have debunked the last thirty years of nutrition information in America."

In the first seventeen minutes, Lustig calmly drops facts like precision bombs:

- As a society, we all weigh *twenty-five pounds more* than our counterparts did twenty-five years ago.
- The world is now experiencing an epidemic of obese *six-month-olds*.
- Even as our total fat consumption has gone down, our obesity has continued to *accelerate*.
- The combination of caffeine and salt in soda is purposefully designed by soda companies to *make you drink more*.
- Simply drinking one soda per day is worth fifteen and a half pounds of fat gain per year.
- Americans are currently consuming *sixty-three pounds per person* of high-fructose corn syrup per year.

But it isn't until minute twenty that Lustig throws down the gauntlet:

"My charge before the end of tonight is to demonstrate that *fructose is a poison*."

That's right—a *poison*. And fructose is in sugar—*all* kinds of sugar.

I was hooked. I was astounded. High-fructose corn syrup is bad? Well, sure. We all suspected that anyway. Table sugar too? Um...*okay*. But *honey*? Maple syrup? Agave? *Fruit juice?* Yep. Yep. Yep.

What the hell was going on here? Why, with his charts and graphs and soda company conspiracy theories, was this guy seeming to make so much *sense*? And if it made so much sense, why hadn't we ever heard this information before? Fruit juice is *poison*? What happened to "fruit juice is *health food*"? And "honey is good for you because it's *natural*"? Why not just tell us everything we've ever been told about nutrition is fundamentally *wrong*? It reminded me of that part in the movie *Sleeper* when the guy who's been asleep for two hundred years starts requesting wheat germ and organic honey, and his doctors remark that thinking those things were healthy is "precisely the opposite of what we now know to be true." Could it be that our entire culture has become one great big Woody Allen joke?

Was it really true, as Lustig put it in one interview, that our culture was the modern-day equivalent of an opium den? Everywhere I looked, I realized, people were sick; they were overweight, they were obese, and they were unhappy. Everywhere I looked, I realized, there was sugar in all its myriad guises. Could it be that we were really all just addicts sucking away at our soda-straw hookahs, never making the obvious connection between our "drug" of choice and our rapidly declining health? Most of all, the question I couldn't let go of was: in a society as awash in sugar as ours, how *do* you escape from the opium den? Is it even *possible*?

And then I got an idea. An awful idea. Right then, I got a wonderful, awful idea.

What would happen… I wondered.

If.

I thought about it. And thought about it. I couldn't stop thinking about it. It was as if someone had spilled seltzer on the keyboard of my brain: it was sizzling and spitting and making very strange humming noises that only I could hear. Forget a lightbulb above my head; this was an acetylene *torch*. I realized I had better talk to Steve.

If my husband thought I was completely out of my mind, he hid it well. Instead of being horrified or dismissive, he seemed intrigued if a bit apprehensive.

"*A whole year* without sugar?" he wondered aloud. "Hmm."

Yes. This was my idea: the whole family—myself, my husband Steve, *and* our two daughters, ages six and eleven—we would not eat added sugar for a *whole year*. The more I thought about it, the more sense it seemed to make. Why *not shun sugar*, specifically fructose? Find out how hard it really would be?

I was a writer, after all, and I had been looking for a new project to focus on. I had seen *Super Size Me*, and I had read *Animal Vegetable Miracle* and *Julie and Julia*—all projects by people who might not have been experts per se, but who had an overwhelming desire to do something unusual, something out of the mainstream—and perhaps, in the process, come to some unforeseen conclusions about themselves and the culture we live in. They all involved food. They all involved a proscribed time period. That was key: I knew I'd never get everyone on board for this project unless the experiment had a definitive beginning and a definitive ending. A yearlong timeline was long enough to really *mean* something, to represent a true commitment and shift to a whole different way of doing things. Maybe even long enough to see some potential changes in ourselves develop. Would our temperaments change? Our waistlines? Our blood work? Our palates? And yet, still, it wasn't *forever*.

At that point, I knew we didn't go so much as a single day in our house without having some form of sugar or other, perhaps not even a single meal, so this experiment was pretty much guaranteed to wreak all kinds of unpredictable havoc with our lives. I loved it.

I would start a blog and write about what happened, the day-to-day events that were bound, I thought, to be interesting or surprising, or frustrating or funny. The writer in me loved the idea of searching out the answers one by one like a kitchen-cupboard Sherlock Holmes. Not just for ourselves, but for others as curious as I was. Had anyone done this before? Could we really do it? What would actually happen? Would we all be abjectly miserable for twelve months? Would we all grow thin and haggard for lack of cheerful sweetness in our diet? Would we develop superhuman levels of health and agility, able to leap tall boxes of Bran Flakes in a single bound? Would we secretly hoard candy in our shoes and cupcakes in our sock drawers? And oh, God, what about *Halloween*? And *Christmas*??

Well, I reasoned: *There's only one way to find out.*

———

Now I can hear you saying, "But wait a minute! That was quick. Didn't you put up a fight for your beloved sugar? Didn't you go for at least a *dip* in the river of Denial?"

Well, perhaps I should back up.

Up until the year of the experiment, we—myself, my husband, and our two daughters, Greta and Ilsa—were a *fairly* normal family when it came to food, I think. Perhaps a bit on the liberal, organic, dirt-worshipping side, but nevertheless, still *fairly* middle of the road. We ate meat. We liked snacks. We liked desserts. When the circus came to town, we'd throw caution to the wind and purchase big, fluffy balls of electric-pink cotton candy despite all our better judgment. Life is short, I reasoned, and although I have my requisite worried-Vermont-mom concerns, (hormone-free beef? GMO corn? pesticides in the potatoes?), I tried to keep them in check. I didn't want my kids growing up being afraid to *live.*

We had come to this particular, carefully balanced point after a fair amount of dietary experimentation, especially before the kids were born and we had time for such nonsense. I had been a steadfast vegetarian of varying shades and colors over a period of two decades, and my husband had dabbled in the vegetal arts as well, although rumor has it he did it to impress a certain girlfriend who turned out to be me.

Once we were good and married, Steve began, over time, to reveal his carnivorous side. I did most of the cooking around the house, so vegetarian still remained the house rule, if not always that of its inhabitants.

What I didn't realize when Steve and I wed was that I was inheriting a family nutrition expert as well: Bill, Steve's father. Perhaps *expert* isn't quite the right word for someone who changed his mind so frequently, and sometimes radically. *Obsessive* might be closer. He was a man possessed by the idea of superior health and the use of nutrition as a means to that end.

Bill, who passed away a few years ago, was a vegetarian before people even knew what that was, back when health food stores were fringe operations frequented and operated by folks who still thought communes might be a really good idea. But Bill Schaub was no long-haired hippy; he was a trim, clean-shaven lawyer who rose over a period of decades to become Regional Director of the National Labor Relations Board and be conferred the rank of Meritorious Executive in the Senior Executive Service by President Bill Clinton. I try to picture him walking into the Toledo-area granola shop in his fresh-pressed suit, his aftershave clashing with the smell of patchouli and wheat grass.

In one favorite Bill Schaub story, he grew a mustache. (Of course he did! It was the seventies!) This development coincided with the peak of his interest in the nutritional value of mangos and his decision to import boxes of the fruit himself, which of course resulted in his brown mustache turning bright orange from the sheer volume of fruit that passed his lips.

There are lots of Bill Schaub anecdotes like this, illustrating not only his passion and single-mindedness when it came to the subject of nutrition and food, but also his mercurial nature—one year it was mangos, the next it would be something else. When we had Greta, while other people were sending us *The Poky Little Puppy* and *There's a Wocket in my*

Pocket!, Bill sent us *Disease-Proof Your Child: Feeding Kids Right*. He had a subscription to *Dr. Shelton's Hygienic Review* and *The China Study* was his idea of some light evening reading. The first time I heard about the Atkins diet was when Bill went on it. After thirty years as a vegetarian, he woke up one morning and would suddenly eat nothing but meat, breakfast, lunch, and dinner.

Steve is his father's son and inherited from him not only an attentive attitude toward food and nutrition, but also the ability to endure strange and restrictive diets. He is also a former marine, and that generally means he can be his own best drill instructor. I've watched him try water diets, egg and meat diets, vegetable diets, various vitamin regimens—you get the idea. So far I've been able to talk him out of fasting, which Bill turned to also—once for a distressing period of over two weeks (albeit in a supervised setting).

The one diet Steve and I tried together was the MacDougall Plan, which, as I recall it now, was comprised primarily of eating brown rice with brown rice on top. I wandered around all day dreaming about grilled cheese sandwiches and yogurt. "Have an apple!" Steve would cheerily suggest when I complained of feeling hungry in between meals. I lasted about two days.

So, between Steve and his father, I now knew more than I ever wanted to know about food fads and nutrition crazes. I was tired of extreme eating that was supposed to be The Answer to everything from having more energy to curing cancer. I wanted my family to eat healthily but in a way that was psychologically sustainable.

FEAR OF FOOD
– BY STEPHEN SCHAUB –

Food and I have always had a very complicated relationship, in part due to my father's obsession with diet and health, so when Eve began talking about A Year of No Sugar for our family, it sent my mind and emotions into a bit of a dark flashback to my own confused childhood with regards to food.

My father was a very intellectual man and always looking for the perfect diet that would provide a life of good health free of disease, most of all cancer. Some of my earliest childhood memories of my dad are of him fasting, eating LOTS of lettuce, and taking my brother and I to the local health food store for fresh fruits and vegetables. The time he took us to see *Star Wars* at the movie theater, I wasn't very excited at first, because I figured he was probably taking us to a lecture on the virtue of broccoli or something. He bought reverse osmosis water in enormous jugs and talked about the benefits of shark cartilage. He tried weird hobbies no one had ever heard of like yoga and organic gardening. Over the years, his diet slowly ranged the entire map of food extremism as he read new books and nutrition literature: one day he'd be eating only vegetables and standing on his head in the living room, the next he'd be eating only meat and talking about Russian strength training. This was my dad.

My mother, on the other hand, loves snack foods and always worked very hard to be a buffer from my father's sometimes-obsessive dietary diatribes. While Dad did his own thing, for the rest of us she cooked regular, Midwestern meals: meat, vegetable, starch. Her chocolate pudding desserts as an after-school snack were loved by both my brother and me, but we knew they needed to be finished, without a trace of them in the fridge before my father was home from work. Don't get me wrong, my father was not some food-controlling tyrant, but rather he felt he could save us from all the bad stuff out there, from the health consequences a poor diet would create in our lives. It was love in the form of carrots and lettuce.

So when my father was diagnosed with cancer at age fifty-nine, I could not help but feel that so much of his life had been built on a belief that had betrayed him. Good food makes you healthy. The sacrifice of not eating a particular snack or type of food would be outweighed by a better quality of life and longevity. Had he been wrong? Despite all his efforts, all his studying of nutrition and all the dedication to one plan of eating or another, he nonetheless came down with the one disease he feared most.

Even after the diagnosis, though, my father refused to give up on his belief in the power of nutrition and extreme eating, which was probably very important, since his belief in the healing power of modern medicine was shaky at best. He listened to his doctors to a point but put his true faith in what he ultimately decided was the perfect anticancer diet: a grueling regime of liquefied lettuce, large slices of watermelon, and the occasional plain, baked sweet potato.

Perhaps it really did help prolong his life—after the initial diagnosis of stage four non-Hodgkin's lymphoma he would live another five years—but if so, it was at a tremendous cost.

This new diet would require an effort beyond all the others which had preceded it and would alter our relationship with him for the rest of his life. During these years, visits were difficult. Meal preparation took a significant portion of every day: shopping for, washing, drying, and finally juicing fields of fresh lettuce into kryptonite green drinks. Traveling and eating out were all but impossible. We supported his need to have a sense of control over his own life and made the best of a very difficult situation—what else could we do? We loved him.

In the end, like so many who suffer cancer, my father died a horrible death. I will always feel sadness thinking about the separation from his family members and friends that his relationship with food created throughout his life.

So it was with this history rooted deep within me that I heard my wife's suggestion with a sense of both curiosity and panic. Eve is a very, very levelheaded woman. I knew for her to suggest such a radical idea, especially with her knowledge of my father and his longtime history of food fears, meant that this was terribly important to her. We have had a strong marriage—at that point thirteen years and counting. For even longer than that time, she has been my best friend, my partner, and my greatest advocate for my work as an artist. How could I not support her now?

After weeks of talking and conferring with professionals that we were not going to wreck our children's childhoods or create a fear of food in their lives—as still exists to some degree in mine—I cautiously gave my vote to do the project. Eve was already full-steam ahead.

———————

Meanwhile, we nonetheless found ourselves members of a larger community increasingly rife with dietary restrictions, both voluntary and otherwise. Unlike when I was growing up, when it seemed to my kid-eyes as if pretty much everyone ate pretty much everything, these days we have many, many hyphenated friends: we have gluten-free friends for whom I never remember to leave the noodles out of the soup. We have organic-only friends who raise and slaughter fifty-two chickens every fall—one for every week of the year. We have vegan friends and local-only friends and nut-free friends and lactose-intolerant friends. We have friends for whom I can't figure out what is left for them to eat but cardboard and paste. Sometimes it's voluntary, other times decidedly not, and most often the necessity of such restrictions falls murkily somewhere in between, as in, "No, I haven't been diagnosed celiac/lactose intolerant/digestively opposed to purple, but I just *feel* so much better when I avoid wheat/cheese/eggplant and grapes." You can understand why all the etiquette experts are repeatedly queried by anxious hostesses about how to deal with so many different potential guests who

1. can't eat
2. won't eat
3. would rather be boiled alive than have it suggested they consider eating

...so many different things.

And did I mention we live in Vermont? Home to back-to-the-landers, experimental-living-arrangements, and more massage therapists than you can shake a stick at? I have seen more god-awful things put forth on plates in the name of healthful sustenance than I care to recount here, but suffice it to say that the jicama-and-zucchini salad is *never* as good as you hope it will be. I'll never forget when Greta was little and a fellow mother was incidentally describing how her kids were playing with their regular breakfast of "tofu and carrots," and I had trouble listening to the rest of the story. *Seriously?* I thought. *Tofu and carrots* for breakfast? Should we all just have our taste buds commit hara-kari *right now?*

Then again, because Vermont is still part of America, the *other* side of the spectrum is also everywhere around us too; you could call it modern-day Caligulanism. Greta, at age eleven, regularly came home from school regaling me with tales of her classmates' trips to Pizza Hut and McDonald's and ice cream for dessert every night. I myself had been dismayed to witness kids bringing armloads of Lunchables and Snackwell's and whole liters of Mountain Dew on school field trips. One day at the supermarket, I stared in open-mouthed horror at the cart of the woman in front of me who was buying nothing but sugar in a variety of different colorful packages: soda, sports drinks, Kool-Aid mix, pudding cups, frosted cereals. Though we lived in the same town and she had a small child in tow, just like me, I marveled at how different our two carts could possibly be, as if we came from two different *planets*. Or species.

So, long before the fateful day when I sat down and began to watch Dr. Lustig's medi-mercial, I had already given the question of how one should best eat a considerable, really *inordinate*, amount of thought. What is the best path to follow, in between eating everything and eating nothing? Where did our family fall, between the McDonald's folks and the tofu-and-carrots-for-breakfast folks? Between worrying all the time and never worrying at all? Many was the time I had felt that there were *so* many different parameters that I felt morally, ethically, and nutritionally compelled to obey that following them all at once would likely mean making our family's diet a full-time unpaid job. Organic? Free-range? Hormone-free? Local? Eco-friendly packaging? Non-genetically modified? Free of laboratory-born, unpronounceable ingredients? And what about pasteurization versus raw? Were we even allowed to *care* whether it tasted good? The more we know, the better off we are *supposed* to be, but the unvarnished reality was that the more I knew, the more frustrated I was guaranteed to be at the supermarket.

I had been looking for the Occam's razor solution (to badly paraphrase, "The simplest answer is usually the correct one") to the problem of modern eating. After reading Michael Pollan counsel with Zen-like simplicity, "Eat Food. Not Too Much. Mostly Plants," I decided this was the closest I'd heard to something sustainable that made sense. From that point on, I positioned myself as a concerned mom who cares about what her family eats *within reason*. If the supermarket didn't carry free-range meat, I'd grudgingly buy the regular chicken. If I couldn't find nice-looking apples that were organic, I'd buy the local ones that weren't. I'd visit the farmer's market and try hard to buy local, but I would surely buy a jalapeño from Mexico if it meant I could make my turkey chili that night. You couldn't be Mary Practically Perfect Poppins all the time, so I gave it my best shot and then let it go. You might call it the "happy medium, dammit" approach.

And then, one day, I became aware of a disturbance in the natural order of things.

I distinctly remember the first time it came up. We

were planning Greta's fifth birthday party, and one of the mothers had asked about the ingredients of my cupcakes. I rattled them off easily, confident there would be no objections to my from-scratch home baking: flour, sugar, baking powder, vanilla—

"Oh, *vanilla*," she stopped me. "Ariella can't have vanilla. It has corn syrup in it. It makes her *crazy*."

"Corn syrup?" *Really? What an odd thing to bother worrying about*, I thought. Although the mom assured me that it was in *"everything"* and that her daughter became erratic and hyperactive anytime she consumed anything with this ingredient in it, I was silently skeptical. After all, this was not some Day-Glo impostor from the "bakery" aisle at the supermarket; this was *home* baked! Made with *love*! As far as I was concerned, homemade food *was* health food. Period. Wasn't that what Michael Pollan had effectively said?

Later on, I came to realize that what my friend had been talking about was, in fact, *high-fructose* corn syrup. And about three milliseconds after making that connection I began to notice that, well, yeah, HFCS *was* everywhere, actually. Pretty much every time I read an ingredient list on a box, *there it would be*, like an annoying ex-boyfriend who can't take a hint already. *Huh. Well, that is a little weird*, I thought. And then suddenly, out of nowhere, high-fructose corn syrup was coming up in conversations, people were talking about it in wide-eyed, "Oh, but haven't you *heard*?" tones. HFCS, it seemed, was fast becoming the Area 51 of the food world: prone to controversy, conspiracy theories, and eventual dismissal by most of the couldn't-be-bothered population at large. Yet, right then, at that moment, it seemed that the "couldn't be bothereds" were shrinking, and the conspiracy theorists were gaining. Overnight, commercials and magazine ads appeared featuring attractive moms duking it out over whether containing high-fructose corn syrup *meant* anything. Suddenly, products began touting their lack of it on packaging: "Made with Real Cane Sugar!" which really meant: "No Mysterious, Chemically-Sounding Potentially-Maybe Bad Stuff!" Entire websites cropped up devoted to promoting high-fructose corn syrup's nutritional evil or innocence.

It seemed that the reason people were so quickly and easily freaked out was based exclusively on the fact that we had suddenly—as a culture—all come to the simultaneous realization how *in everything* this stuff was. Americans can put up with a *lot* of stuff, as long as they have at least the illusion of a choice in the matter; here, the supermarket illusion of choice had been revealed to be no choice at all—there was no escaping demonic-sounding "HFCS." Ooo! It was as if the food industry had made our decisions for us, overnight, at some questionable warehouse on the outskirts of town, and we were all waking up the next day realizing it after the fact. They seemed to be saying to us: oh, so you *want* to buy bread at the supermarket? Crackers? Salad dressing? You say you're too *busy* to make these things yourself at home? Well, we're businessmen; we can be reasonable. Listen—we're gonna make you an offer you can't refuse…

I was skeptical, though. Just like acai berries are magically *good* (never mind why), high-fructose corn syrup is magically *bad* (never mind why)? Yet, like many concerned consumers, I just didn't like the *sound* of it. What the hell *was* it? Why was it everywhere? Why was it so hard to find crackers or cereal or even *bread* without it? How much of this stuff were we eating, anyway, without ever having realized it? And what was wrong with using sugar or honey or something, you know, more *natural?* So, based on this oh-so-highly-scientific analysis of the facts, our family abruptly stopped buying products containing high-fructose corn syrup. There were still plenty of other things to buy, and it only entailed a *bit* more label reading. Michael Pollan advised buying food products with no more than five ingredients anyway, so we tried to stick to that too. We made our bread at home with local honey; we bought raw sugar for homemade cookies and pies. And once again, we felt like good people who cared about what our family ate.

For a while.

CHAPTER 3

A SWEET POISON

And so it came to pass that our author watched the ninety-minute video by Dr. Robert Lustig. And the words of the prophet burned with the light of truth in her eyes. She was not blinded, nay, but she was truly perturbed. And she saw with a new vision, that the vile substance which, yea, had brought pestilence and disease in its wake, was indeed everywhere. And she was totally freaked out.

Here's the thing. I'm never going to be confused for a doctor or a nutritionist, or anybody who has credentials of any sort, really. I'm pretty much *not* the person you'd ask to explain any medical theory of any kind. It's okay—I *know* I'm not the next Sanjay Gupta, and I can live with that.

But our family had decided to *not eat added sugar for a year* (the parameters of which I promise to explain in detail in the chapters to come), and it's important to understand that this wasn't simply a whim or a fun, kicky idea or even a masochistic challenge. Rather, it was really and truly the result of being *convinced*, in a fundamental way, that **sugar is everywhere, it's making us all fat and sick, and almost no one realizes it**—and then wanting to do something about it. Something *real* that would demonstrate to us, and others, what it entails to get away from sugar.

You know the commercial where the one smart, concerned-looking mom is making the other mom feel really stupid for avoiding high-fructose corn syrup? "Whether it's corn sugar or cane sugar, your body can't tell the difference" is the industry tagline. The funny thing is, they are right.

In "Sugar: The Bitter Truth," Dr. Robert Lustig explains that, contrary to popular opinion, high-fructose corn syrup is *not worse* for you than ordinary table sugar; it's simply *equally bad*. The reason? Because of the *fructose*. And here is where the argument becomes tricky. When you stop talking about sugar and start talking about *fructose*, and bringing out words like *ghrelin* and *leptin* and *antidisestablishmentarianism*, people start to glaze over and get fidgety. Tell them that *fat* makes you *fat*, or *carbs* make you *fat*, or foods that are *beige* make you *fat*, and people listen, remember, and believe. But tell them that fructose fails to suppress ghrelin? Not so much.

Consequently, what follows is my best attempt to summarize the not-always-so-very-straightforward argument as to what sugar (fructose) does in your body (bad things) and why it is such a scary thing (it's killing us). As our project began to unfold, I would come to rely heavily on the arguments of two important no-sugar advocates who understand biochemistry a lot better than I ever will: the aforementioned Dr. Robert Lustig, professor of Pediatric Endocrinology at UC San Francisco, and David Gillespie, author of a very interesting book published in Australia titled *Sweet Poison*. (Statistics from other sources such as the CDC or JAMA are cited.)

So without further ado, let's unveil our Handy Dandy Cheat Sheet:

How Fructose Makes You Fat and Sick

1. *All* sugar contains fructose.
2. Fructose does not satisfy hunger, *so you eat more food than your body needs*.
3. Fructose may not be used by any of the cells in our body, except the liver.
4. In processing fructose, the liver produces bad things: **uric acid** and **fatty acids**.
5. Too much **uric acid** causes:
   > Gout
   > Hypertension
6. Too many **fatty acids** cause:
   > Nonalcoholic Fatty Liver Disease (NAFLD)
   > Cardiovascular Disease (CVD)
   > Insulin Resistance & Type 2 Diabetes
   > Obesity
7. The clustering of two or more of the four conditions above is called **Metabolic Syndrome**. Virtually unheard of only a few decades ago, *one in five Americans* suffers from it today.
8. Additionally, circulating **fatty acids** have been proven to speed the growth of *cancer cells*.
9. Consumption of fructose has risen *341 percent* in the last century and continues to climb.
10. So what do you call something that our body has no need for and that, when we take it in, creates toxic by-products in our bodies resulting in debilitation, disease, and untimely death? Well, doctors call that a *poison*.

That's a lot to swallow all at one time, isn't it? But let's take it point by point:

1. *All* **sugar contains fructose**: Name a sugar, any sugar: table sugar, high-fructose corn syrup, maple syrup, molasses, agave, evaporated cane syrup, honey, fruit juice, powdered sugar, brown sugar, crystalline fructose, and so on. In each, the sweetness has been extracted from the original sources, be it fruit, beets, maple sap, honeycomb, or sugar cane.

In most sweeteners, the sweetness comes from a combination of both glucose and fructose.[3] Percentages of fructose in sweeteners vary: both table sugar and HFCS are roughly half fructose, half glucose, whereas supposedly healthy agave contains up to *90 percent* fructose. Now here's an important part: Glucose is Good. Glucose is what your body, and all living things, use to transport energy through the body and is what Lustig refers to as "the energy of life." It is the inability of the body to access that *good* glucose that results in diabetes, but more on that in a minute.

2. **Fructose does not satisfy hunger** *so you eat more food than your body needs.* Once upon a time, our bodies only encountered fructose in tiny amounts from seasonal fruit. Not only was that fruit fairly hard to come by, but lots of fiber and micronutrients necessarily came with it, thereby helping balance any potential negative effect of that small amount of fructose.

Problems would only begin to arise about seven thousand years ago, when humans got a bright idea. One day, after

---

[3]With the exception of crystalline fructose, which is composed entirely of fructose.

enjoying sucking on stalks of sugar cane for centuries, people decided to try *extracting* the best part. The resulting sweet sap became wildly popular of course, so much so that folks who didn't have ready access to the sugar cane began experimenting with other things toward a similar end, such as extracting the juice from a particularly sweet variety of beets. Nonetheless, these were labor-intensive processes and sweeteners would remain prohibitively expensive for some time. It wouldn't be until the industrial age that sugar would suddenly and irrevocably begin a downward spiral in price, and correspondingly, people began adding it to more and more things. Finally, in 1975, HFCS arrived on the scene as the ultimate cheap ingredient—made from government-subsidized corn and used as filler in everything from lunch meats and soup to baby formula.

Unfortunately for us, however, fructose does a very funny thing biochemically speaking, something we couldn't have begun to notice until huge volumes of people began consuming huge amounts of the stuff over long periods of time. Fructose, as it turns out, exploits a loophole in your body's carefully orchestrated ballet of hormones: fructose does not suppress ghrelin (the hunger hormone) *nor* does it stimulate insulin or leptin (the full-feeling hormone). You get the fructose's *calories*, of course, but *you are still as hungry as if you hadn't eaten them*. So you keep eating.

Here's a scary instance of what this really means in practice: studies have shown that a teenager who drinks a soda before a meal *will eat more* at that meal,[4] not less—and in our

[4]Robert Lustig, "Sugar: The Bitter Truth," YouTube video, 1:29:28, University of California Television, posted by UCTV, July 30, 2009, http://www.youtube.com/watch?v=dBnniua6-oM

culture, of course, that likely means you will eat *more sugar*. Talk about a vicious cycle.

Now imagine if our country's food system were dominated by eating, say, cardboard. We all found cardboard unbelievably delicious, so we crushed it up and put it in *everything*. Only trouble being: cardboard isn't something our body needs or wants, so it doesn't register with our hormones—it doesn't make us feel full. So we keep eating it and eating it. Our bodies have to do something with all that cardboard, so we all start growing "cardboard bellies," all the while wondering why we are always so hungry, why it is always so hard to lose weight. This is what fructose is like.

Except it's worse. Because—

3. Fructose may not be used by any of the cells in our body, except the liver. Another key indicator that our body wasn't built for lots of fructose consumption is the fact that we have no receptors for it: no cells have "Welcome, Fructose!" mats on their doorsteps…quite the contrary. Most of them have hand-lettered signs reading: "Fructose Not Welcome Here" and "We Don't Speak Fructose." Consequently, while only 20 percent of calories from glucose end up in the liver, the rest having been absorbed and used along the way in our digestive system, *all* fructose—100 percent of its calories—must go to the liver to be processed, just like those of toxins. And just like with toxins, there in the liver, many things happen—all of them bad, as we shall see.

Lustig compares the effects of fructose to those of a toxin we know and love: ethanol (alcohol). A comparison of the symptoms of chronic alcohol consumption to those of chronic fructose consumption reveals that they share *eight out of twelve* disorders, fun things like pancreatitis and dyslipidemia. He concludes that "fructose is ethanol without the buzz" and asserts that giving your kid a soda—*or* juice—is the metabolic equivalent of giving your kid a *beer*. So, how scary is that?

4. In processing fructose, the liver produces *bad things*: uric acid and fatty acids. As with toxins, when the liver has to process fructose, it creates some not-so-terrific things to have in your body. In great enough amounts, those not-so-terrific things cause specific, identifiable problems that get progressively worse over time. For example...

5. Too much uric acid causes:

Gout—Characterized by attacks of acute inflammatory arthritis, gout used to be known as the "disease of kings" or "the gentleman's disease" because primarily the wealthy suffered from it. Remember: sugar was expensive up until only about one hundred years ago.

Hypertension—Uric acid blocks an important liver enzyme that is your body's in-house blood-pressure lowerer. According to a 2010 report by the CDC, *25 percent* of the total U.S. population over age eighteen is diagnosed with hypertension.[5]

6. Too many fatty acids cause:

Nonalcoholic Fatty Liver Disease—Cirrhosis of the liver: it's not just for alcoholics anymore! NAFLD,[6] just like

---

[5]Schiller, J.S., J.W. Lucas, B.W. Ward, and J.A. Peregoy, "Summary Health Statistics for U.S. Adults: National Health Interview Survey, 2010," *Vital Health and Statistics*, 10(252), 2012, U.S. Department of Health and Human Services, http://www.cdc.gov/nchs/data/series/sr_10/sr10_252.pdf

[6]aka, nonalcoholic steatohepatitis

the alcoholic version, results from the accumulation of fatty tissue in the liver that creates inflammation and scar tissue. Previously unheard of, *non*alcoholic fatty liver disease was identified and named in the 1980s,[7] yet it is estimated that *up to 24 percent* of the U.S. population now suffers from it.[8]

Cardiovascular Disease—Hypertension, Angina, Heart Attack, Stroke…know anyone with one of these? Unfortunately, CVD is all the rage these days, accounting for *one out of every four* American deaths in 2009.[9] Heart disease is the leading killer in the U.S. today.

But here's a counterintuitive news flash: *fat doesn't cause heart disease.* Sugar does. In one particularly illuminating moment in "Bitter Truth," Lustig explains that there are not one but *two* forms of what we call "bad" cholesterol or LDLs (low-density lipoproteins): "large buoyant" and "small dense." When your LDLs are measured, they measure both kinds together, but in fact, it is *only* the small, dense LDLs that get stuck in the walls of our blood vessels, beginning the formation of plaque and causing cardiovascular disease. Guess what raises the large buoyant LDLs, the *good* LDLs? Dietary fat.

---

[7]Ludwig J., T.R. Viggiano, D.B. McGill, and B.J. Oh. "Nonalcoholic Steatohepatitis: Mayo Clinic Experiences with a Hitherto Unnamed Disease—Abstract," Mayo Clin Proc. 1980 Jul; 55(7): 434–8, http://www.ncbi.nlm.nih.gov/pubmed/7382552

[8]David Gillespie, *Sweet Poison: Why Sugar Makes Us Fat*, (Australia: Penguin, 2008) 120.

[9]Kenneth D. Kochanek, M.A.; Jiaquan Xu, M.D.; Sherry L. Murphy, B.S.; Arialdi M. Miniño M.P.H.; and Hsiang-Ching Kung, Ph.D., Division of Vital Statistics. "Deaths: Preliminary Data for 2009: National Vital Statistics Reports," *National Vital Statistics Reports* vol. 59, no. 4 (March 16, 2011) U.S. Department of Health and Human Services, http://www.cdc.gov/nchs/data/nvsr/nvsr59/nvsr59_04.pdf

On the other hand, the small dense LDLs? The *bad* guys? Those are raised by carbohydrates. When the low-fat craze of the 1980s hit, and food processors began coming out with low-fat versions of all their products, what carbohydrate did they use to replace the great taste of fat? Why, sugar, of course. So in addition to all the obvious sugar—the soda, the candy bars, the Hostess Fruit Pies—we also have an entire universe of hidden sugar, in things that aren't even sweet and in places you'd never suspect—sugar in our gravy, salad dressings, sauces. Sugar in our tortellini and chicken broth and baby food. The entire middle of the supermarket is an amalgamation of processed foods in packages, boxes, and bags...and most of it contains some form of sugar.[10] This is why, despite the fact that Americans' fat consumption has gone down, our rates of cardiovascular disease have continued to go *up*.

Insulin Resistance & Type II Diabetes—But just like everywhere else in the body, fructose gets no welcome mat in the pancreas either; there are no receptors for fructose on the cells in the pancreas that make insulin. When you consume fructose, the pancreas doesn't know and doesn't care; no corresponding insulin gets released. Instead, those carbohydrate-generated fats start to accumulate in the bloodstream, getting in the way of the acceptance of good glucose by the cells of your body. Unlike fructose, or the circulating fats that fructose eventually results in, your body desperately needs that glucose to continue all its normal functions. "Energy of life," remember?

---

[10]According to a recent count, *eighty percent* of packaged food products contain added sugar. Robert H. Lustig, M.D., *Fat Chance: Beating the Odds Against Sugar, Processed Food, Obesity, and Disease*, (New York: Hudson Street Press, 2012) 234.

Think of insulin as the guy with the key to glucose's new apartment (the cell)—we'll call him Fred. Glucose just *can't* get into its new place without Fred McInsulin's help. But all those circulating fats are getting in the way, jamming up all the major thoroughfares like a rush hour traffic jam, making it harder and harder for the important glucose to get through—eventually resulting in what is called *insulin resistance*. In an attempt to keep the body supplied with fuel—which is there but can't get through—the pancreas, confused, continues to manufacture more and more and *more* insulin. (What happened to Fred? Better send his sister over with another key. Also his cousin and nephew just to be sure.) But the roads are still jammed! No one is getting through—not Fred, not his relatives, not Glucose. Finally, the pancreas either wears out, or the glucose is unable to be used as fuel no matter how much insulin is produced. Voilà! Diabetes Type 2.[11]

This is the unfortunate magic trick fructose has been playing over and over again throughout the sugar-eating world. Whereas in 1900, diabetes was as rare as a hippo with a hernia, today the CDC and the WHO have officially characterized type 2 diabetes as a worldwide *epidemic*.[12]

Obesity—Ah, yes. The word that's on everyone's lips these days. "Why are we all so *fat*?" Western society wonders to itself.

Here, at long last, is the answer: yet another of the many bad things fructose does in the liver is it stimulates something called *de novo lipogenesis*, literally: New Fat Making. Woo-hoo! So, just to recap, not only do you have circulating fat *in* your *arteries*, as a free bonus, you also get to add

---

[11]Gillespie, *Sweet Poison*, 114.

[12]Gillespie, *Sweet Poison*, 115.

*non*circulating fat to your *waistline*. That's two fats for the price of one!

Not coincidentally, a century ago, before sugar got cheap and our consumption went through the roof, a mere one in twenty-five people was clinically obese. Today in the U.S., *one in three* is.[13] Not just fat, mind you; one third of the U.S. population is *obese*.

7. The clustering of two or more of the four conditions above is called *Metabolic Syndrome*. Virtually unheard of only a few decades ago, one in five Americans suffers from *Metabolic Syndrome* today.[14] If you've never heard of Metabolic Syndrome, get ready—by all rights, it should be one of the new buzzwords for the decade, right up there with "tornadic activity" and "fo shizzle."[15] Although the specific criteria can vary depending who you're talking to, in order to be identified as having metabolic syndrome, one would have *more than one* of the conditions listed above…as if having one of them wasn't fun enough.

According to U.S. census data, in 2000, there were an estimated *forty-seven million Americans* living with metabolic syndrome.[16] If we believe the Cleveland Clinic's more recent

---

[13]Gillespie, *Sweet Poison*, 99.

[14]"Diseases and Conditions: Metabolic Syndrome," Cleveland Clinic, http://my.clevelandclinic.org/disorders/metabolic_syndrome/hic_metabolic_syndrome.aspx

[15]For the record, I have no idea what this means.

[16]Ford, Earl S., MD, MPH; Wayne H. Giles, MD, MSc; William H. Dietz, MD, PhD, "Prevalence of the Metabolic Syndrome Among U.S. Adults: Findings from the Third National Health and Nutrition Examination Survey," *The Journal of the American Medical Association*, vol. 287, no. 3 (January 16, 2002), http://jama.ama-assn.org/content/287/3/356

estimate of one in five, that means now there are more than *sixty-two million Americans*[17] living with a condition the term for which was coined as recently as 1977.

8. Additionally, circulating fatty acids have been proven to speed the growth of cancer cells. As if everything we've already mentioned weren't enough reason to run screaming from the sugar-added buffet at our local supermarket, we can add cancer to the mix as well. And not just *any* cancers: three out of the five most common cancers—colorectal, breast, and prostate—as well as one of the most deadly—pancreatic—all have proven correlations with increased sugar intake.[18]

Simply put, cancerous cells consume more glucose than normal cells. Therefore, if you have a heightened blood-glucose level (due to all those lovely circulating fatty acids that interrupt the glucose from getting to your cells) you have a very cancer-cell-friendly environment on your hands.

Sweet Poison author David Gillespie points out some rather startling correlations between consumption of sugar and prostate cancer deaths: when consumption of sugar has gone down, for example due to the wartime shortages of the 1940s, the rates of prostate cancer also drops—*sixty years later*. Then, when sugar became plentiful again? Prostate cancers went up again—sixty years later. The two graphs mimic one another uncannily—a six-decade shadow. Remember: sugar is a *chronic* toxin—give it some time, and it will do some very bad things.

---

[17]Although I have seen other estimates as high as seventy-five million.

[18]Gillespie, *Sweet Poison*, 120.

9. Consumption of fructose has risen *341 percent* in the last century and continues to climb. In the beginning of the 1900s, we consumed about five ounces of fructose per week, or approximately sixteen pounds per person, per year. Today we consume about 140 pounds of sugar, or *70.5 pounds of fructose per person, per year—an increase of 341 percent*. Meanwhile, we're all getting fatter and sicker at an alarming rate, with disease after disease that was virtually unheard of a century ago, each of which directly correlates to the biology of sugar consumption. Coincidence?

Often, the effects of a toxin, such as alcohol, are distressing because of their acute symptoms, the ones which appear right away. But just as detrimental, if not more so, are the things that a toxin can do over the long term. At least with alcohol, we have something of a "warning" system in the acute symptoms, to let us know when we have consumed far too much. There is no such signifier for fructose—unless you count the Pillsbury Doughboy-ification of America as a signifier. It just quietly poisons us for years and years until something gives: Liver? Pancreas? Heart? Cardiovascular system? Pick your necessary organ and fructose will, eventually, poison it to death.

Now, if you're like my mom, right about now you're saying, with some incredulity, "So you're saying everything my doctor has been telling me—everything *all the doctors* have been telling us—*is wrong*? That heart disease *isn't* caused by animal fats? That eating less and exercising *isn't* the key to losing weight? That fruit juice *isn't* health food?"

Well…yeah.

It wouldn't be the first time such a thing has happened, would it? After all—Einstein's Theory of Relativity upended two hundred years of scientific thought. Pretty much everything everyone had thought about the nature of the universe before that turned out to be just...*wrong*. And remember how the world was supposed to be flat? History is full of good, logical, common-sense ideas that turned out to be completely, dramatically, spectacularly *wrong*.

It was this message—the message that sugar was the missing link, the key to the "curse of the Western diet"—that I began to understand the day I watched Dr. Robert Lustig's video on YouTube. And then I couldn't *stop* thinking about it. I thought about it while washing dishes, while picking my kids up at school, while washing my hair in the shower. I especially thought about it in the supermarket and while cooking. My brain was on fire with this idea that our food supply had been adulterated in plain sight. Had I ever considered before that sugar is not required for our body's proper functioning in any way? The fact that the number of obese Americans has not doubled or even tripled in the last hundred years but, in fact, has increased by *seven* times? What do you even *call* that? Septupled?

The facts as Lustig had cited them ran through my brain over and over. Still, could it be a case of circumstantial evidence? Even if it was, it was still pretty *compelling* circumstantial evidence, along the lines of finding the missing cat's collar in the backseat of the dog's car—it may not assure guilt beyond a reasonable doubt, but it su-u-u-u-re didn't look good. Could it really be that we were eating poison every day, buying it in our supermarkets, sprinkling it on our cereal, and pouring it in the drinking glasses of our children? Could that be what was mysteriously making so many Americans— and the citizens of any country foolish enough to adopt the Western diet—so increasingly, incredibly, amazingly, undeniably fat and sick? Could it be that *this* was the Occam's razor, the simplest answer, I had been waiting for?

And thus was born our family's Year of No Sugar.

CHAPTER 4

SUGAR, SUGAR EVERYWHERE

W e should just go home. *Let's just go home,*" Steve said in the voice he uses when he's trying not to be angry and failing.

"We can't go home without at least eating," I objected.

"Well, *there's nowhere for us to eat!*" He was exasperated and losing it, and truthfully, so was I. We were both long past hungry. It was cold and dark, and we were driving around in circles trying to figure out what to do. The movie we had been hoping to make had already started. Fast food restaurants, chain restaurants were *everywhere*, but because we were not eating sugar, there was no place we could eat. This was turning out to be one big bummer of a date night.

As Steve fumed to the point where I suspected steam might emit from his ears, I quietly began to wonder for the first time what effect our Year of No Sugar would have on our marriage. And did I mention this was only *January*?

Originally, our plan for the night had seemed so simple: Panera was right across the way from the movie theater and has been our not-so-fast-food-y fast food of choice for some time. Even if we couldn't eat most of the sandwiches on the menu—we suspected sugar in the bread, sugar in the deli meats, sugar in the condiments—we could surely get a quick *salad*, right?

Well, if I learn anything at all from our Year of No Sugar, it will be to never assume anything ever again. We were delighted to be the only folks at the counter—no line! No waiting! We'd make this movie yet. We ordered two chicken Caesar salads.

"Would you like baguette, apple, or chips with that?" asked the young lady manning the cash register.

"Does the baguette have sugar in it?" my husband asked. The young lady said she could check and proceeded to haul out the large, three-ring binder I now know exists in most chain restaurants on a shelf just under the counter. She paged through the plastic sheets. Yes, it did.

"What about the chicken salad?" I asked. "Would you mind looking that up for us?"

"Oh, it's no problem," she said, paging some more. First she looked up the Caesar dressing. "Dextrose?" she said uncertainly. Oh heck—what was *dextrose*?

"Well, what about just the salad itself, minus the dressing?" I asked. Now there were people waiting behind us. The list of dressing ingredients took up almost an entire typed sheet of paper, and the chicken salad, when she located it, was worse. There were literally *dozens* of ingredients in the "chicken salad." Would it be too much to ask, I wondered, that the ingredients of a salad with chicken be salad and chicken?

We were starting to feel really self-conscious now. The lady at the counter was still being very nice to us, and I felt bad for her, as if we were the two cranky old people who come in at rush hour and hold up the line for twenty minutes trying to ascertain whether there are any poppy seeds in the poppy seed muffins. Steve turned to me, defeated, and said, "There's no way we're making the movie." The thought that we were paying our babysitter fifteen dollars an hour so that we could drive thirty minutes each way to spend our evening reading ingredient lists at a Panera for our date night was, well, depressing.

Meanwhile, she handed us the book to peruse to the side while she helped some other customers, and as I stared at the page of four million ingredients, I realized he was right: no movie—and it seemed, no dinner either. We thanked the young lady, returned the plastic pages, and left feeling beaten.

Now, let's pause a moment to reflect on this. I knew full well that we had brought this problem on *ourselves*. Not being able to find food or *specific* food that fit our parameters of the moment was certainly a First-World problem if there ever was one. Were we going to *starve* to death? No. It's worth noting here that in our culture, we've gotten rather alarmingly *used* to getting what we want pretty much right when we want it. Because of our status as contemporary Americans, we have an abundant supply of sustenance from any number of sources at almost any given moment. You can buy snacks virtually anywhere these days, from Home Depot and Jo-Ann Fabrics to your local gas station or car repair shop. How eye-opening, then, for me to realize how *much* of this abundant "food" was now off the table for us because of our family project. It made me remember that, in the grand scheme of things, refusing food is a luxury we in the First World enjoy and take for granted. We were going to have to reorient our expectations about the world around us and what we could realistically expect from it. We couldn't rely on the corporations or the car shops or even the quick-food establishments anymore—we had to take responsibility for our nourishment in a much more fundamental way.

So here we were: food, food was everywhere, but not a thing to eat. McDonald's, Burger King, Olive Garden, all the usual fast-eating suspects were right there, and Steve and I both acting hungry enough to eat our own arms. Fortunately, after several rounds of driving in circles and sniping at one another, we settled on a local German restaurant, where I was hopeful some sausages would fit the no-sugar bill. After informing the waitress that I couldn't have a meal with sugar as an ingredient, she checked and found that the wiener schnitzel and the noodle side dish did *not* have sugar in them.

Hallelujah! Hallelujah! We would both have that. Oh, and we get soup and salad with our dinners, what soup and what dressing would we like? We asked if the chowder had sugar in it, and Steve asked if the blue cheese dressing had sugar.

"Wait," she said, "you can't have sugar *either*?" Although I had toyed with the possibilities of telling people we had a contagious sugar allergy or avoided sugar for religious reasons, so far I was just asking, as politely as possible, and not explaining very much. I figured, if people assume I have a dietary restriction due to some health concern, they may be far more likely to be accurate and truthful than if they think I'm doing this for a lark—or just to be completely annoying. This works, of course, until Steve asks *too*, in which case my cover is blown and he starts to tell our waitress about our "family project."

"Oh, how *cool*," our waitress enthused, which was very polite of her because I was fairly certain she didn't think it was cool at all. We chatted about the omnipresence of sugar and such for a moment, and how hard it is to avoid sugar entirely. After a minute, she genuinely asked "So...*why*?"

"Well...to see if it can be done," I said, which wasn't *entirely* untrue. Certainly, that was one aspect of it, although I felt like I was lying by omission in leaving out the whole "oh-and-by-the-way-sugar-is-a-chronic-toxin" thing. Although *I* had bought Dr. Lustig's argument hook, line, and sinker, I wasn't well versed enough in the biochemical specifics yet to confidently make the argument to so much as a houseplant. Plus, I'm guessing people tend to get touchy when you start telling them their restaurant serves poison.

As it turned out, all three of the soups on the menu contained sugar, as well as the blue cheese dressing. Of course. Nonetheless we enjoyed our soup-and-salad-less entrees with as much enthusiasm as if we had just discovered a Perrier fountain in the desert. As we drove home, we vowed to be more prepared in the future—and to be much bigger tippers.

A few months before, in the fall, Steve and I had broken the news to the kids. Our girls, Greta, who was ten then, and Ilsa, who was five, were in the backseat of the car as we drove home from a visit to my mother's. Having thought of the idea the previous spring, I had been chomping at the bit for months on end, eager to begin, but I had no interest in doing it *alone*—the whole point to my idea being that the entire family participate. Sure, *one* person can do any ol' crazy-ass thing—eat nails, live in a Redwood tree, go over Niagara Falls in a corset and heels—but a *whole family*? That meant something much greater, would say so much more—*that* was the idea which had me lying awake at night wondering: Could we? But so far Steve had advocated putting it off, wanting to make sure we were really ready—I saw his point. We didn't want to plunge in too fast, right? But the paranoiac in me wondered: Was he stalling? Was he waiting for me to gradually lose steam, hoping I'd eventually forget about it? If I pushed *too* hard, I risked losing his support for the idea, which was pivotal in getting the girls on board. But with the end of the calendar year now approaching, I couldn't wait any longer—I was bursting to commit to a plan, and what better time to begin a yearlong project than January first? Steve and I finally agreed: It would be January first to January first, beginning to end; it would be our Year of No Sugar.

"We're thinking of doing a special project—as a family," I said in my best overly calm, your-parents-are-totally-sane voice. "We are thinking of not eating sugar. For a while."

It took them about six seconds to ascertain that "no sugar" meant no cupcakes, no pie, no Christmas cookies, no Popsicles, no hot cocoa, no maple syrup, no jelly beans, no candy bars, no juice boxes, and no marshmallows. And it took them about three additional seconds to elicit that "a while" meant "a year" in parent-speak, which meant "for*ever*" in kid-speak. And they promptly burst into hysterical tears.

"Well, *that* went well," Steve said.

In my mind, keeping it simple was the key to making our Year of No Sugar a success, both in helping us to stick to

---

[19]I include in this category not just aspartame (NutraSweet), saccharine (Sweet'N Low), and sucralose (Splenda) but also (eventually) all sugar alcohols (xylitol, Maltitol) and Stevia (Truvia). Although these are all sweeteners that do not contain fructose—and Stevia is even "natural," derived from the Stevia plant—they all are suspected of having side effects of greater or lesser severity, ranging from cancer and stroke to headaches and diarrhea. Fun! I decided: thanks, but no thanks.

WHAT "NO SUGAR" MEANS TO ME:

NO:

- white sugar
- brown sugar
- cane sugar
- confectioner's sugar
- high-fructose corn syrup
- crystalline fructose
- molasses
- maple syrup
- honey
- evaporated cane syrup
- agave
- artificial sweeteners of all stripes[19]
- and yes...fruit juice

EXCEPTION #1: As a family we'll pick one dessert to have every month that can contain sugar. If it is your birthday that month, you get to pick the dessert.

EXCEPTION #2: Every family member gets to pick one exception *for themselves* that contains a *small* amount of sugar.

EXCEPTION #3: The Birthday Party Rule, for the kids only. If you are surrounded by a roomful of kids all simultaneously having the same dessert, the decision whether to have it is up to you.

it and in communicating it to others. It didn't take long for Steve and me to lay down the few ground rules that would govern the year. We would, however, spend the rest of the year fine-tuning the details, as we came upon new information and new, unusual ingredients.

The concept *was* simple: We were *not eating added sugar.* If an item contained sugar as an ingredient, no matter how minuscule the amount, we would not eat it—this avoided any slippery-slope concerns. What did we mean by "added" sugar? Naturally occurring sugar—such as that contained in a piece of fruit—was fine, containing as it did all the beneficial fiber and micronutrients, and naturally limited the amount we ate—you'd get full before you could eat enough fructose to worry about.

But, in the interest of family harmony and not being the subject of a future exposé on what subhumanly crappy parents we were, we would have some exceptions too, number one being: as a family, we would pick *one dessert per month* to have which contained sugar. If it was your birthday that month, you got to pick the dessert. We had all kinds of fun with this one, and it was especially interesting to watch how our attitude toward this "once per month" treat evolved over time…but more on that later.

Secondly, and inspired by Barbara Kingsolver's book *Animal Vegetable Miracle* in which her family ate locally for one year, we used her family's "one exception per person" rule. This would apply to a particular food, not a type of sugar or a category of food. For example, "powdered sugar" or "cookies" would *not* be possible exceptions; "ketchup" or "mayonnaise" would be.

We chose our personal exceptions with little hesitation.

I knew that wine contained a comparatively tiny amount of fructose,[20] but to be completely on the up-and-up, and not have to forgo wine for an entire year, I officially made it my exception. I was interested to get as far away from sugar as I could, so I figured it would be good not to have a truly "sweet" exception. I also figured there would be days in the year ahead when a glass of wine would be sorely needed.

As for Steve, as long as I have known him he's been a bit of a coffee and soda addict—at any given moment, if he wasn't drinking one, he likely was having the other. Diet Dr Pepper was his sweet beverage of choice—and consequently this became his exception. (Although Diet Dr Pepper doesn't actually contain sugar, artificial sweeteners were also off the table for our Year—see footnote above.)

I encouraged (strong-armed?) the girls into choosing jam as their joint exception. Amazingly, they didn't complain. Maybe they bought my argument that we'd get a lot of mileage out of this: school-lunch peanut butter sandwiches and breakfast toast, etc., or maybe they were just resigned to Mommy's new role as dietary dictator. At home, this meant the girls got Polaner All Fruit Jam, which is sweetened with fruit juice. Compared to most jams, it is not terribly sweet.

The third exception dealt specifically with the kids. Because the kids bring their lunches to school, I am in charge of a good ninety percent of what the kids get in terms of food on a regular basis. However, I realized very quickly that when the kids were out in the world—at school *besides* lunchtime, at

---

[20]According to the United States Department of Agriculture's National Nutrient Database for Standard Reference (http://ndb.nal.usda.gov/ndb/foods/show/4116), an average five-ounce glass of red wine contains 0.91 grams of total sugars. It is not broken down further into glucose and fructose.

birthday parties and playdates—that they would be making their own decisions about what they would and would not put in their own mouths. Rather than giving them reason to sneak behind Mom and Dad's back—and encouraging a distrust dynamic that I was loathe to consider—I decided to welcome and incorporate this aspect of individuality into the project. Each kid would have autonomy outside the house, when parents were not there, to make their own decisions about what to eat. I liked to call this the "Birthday Party Rule": if she were at a birthday party, she could decide whether or not to have a piece of cake. If she were at school and they served hot chocolate, she could decide whether or not to have the hot chocolate. The only condition was they had to *tell* me about it—no guilt, no repercussions.

Instead of hiding treats, therefore, our daughters were encouraged to tell us about them as part of our broader family conversation about sugar—it became almost a contest to see who of the four of us could come home with the most outrageous sugar story. This worked extremely well to the point that I became startlingly more aware of just how *many* sugary treats kids are offered on a daily basis from a wide variety of sources: from local businesses and other parents to teachers, the school, and after-school programs. I was also surprised that *sometimes* the kids voluntarily chose to stick with our No Sugar program, even when it was completely up to them. Will wonders never cease?

Likewise, I encouraged Greta, who was old enough to do so, to keep a journal of her experiences. I assured her the journal was *entirely* up to her. She could choose to share it with others or not; she could write in it what she wished. I hoped this would not only give me a different window into her personal experience of the project (if she chose to share it with me) but also give her an outlet for difficult feelings the project was sure to inspire: guilt, frustration, anger, feeling weird and left out. She was, after all, on the verge of teenager-hood—these feelings were bound to be cropping up sooner or later anyway, with or without Mommy's crazy sugar project.

Today we officially started the "NO! Eat Sugar Project."
I'm so worried about this. I know my friends already
think I'm kind of weird. OH right—you don't know
anything about me. First off, my family takes really good
care of me.

Secondly, you need to know my family eats really
healthy and some of my friends think that's somewhat
crazy. I mean, we don't eat Doritos or at fast food places.
Like for instance, I've never been to McDonald's and I've
also never been to Subway.[21] Still my sister likes to look at
a McDonald's playground (nearby). I have to admit I am
tempted but not really wanting to go.

—from Greta's journal

Originally, and out of desperation, I attempted to add a fourth exception to the list, to wit: "Fruit juice may be an ingredient

---

[21]Although Subway does a good job marketing itself as the "healthy fast food," even prior to the No Sugar year, I have never been convinced. This suspicion would be confirmed for me as we came to learn how much hidden sugar can be in sandwiches: in the bread, in the glazes the meats are cooked in, in the condiments and dressings.

if actual fruit is *also* an ingredient," which would've enabled me to buy things as varied as health-food-store gummy bears and apple sausages. Steve called me on that one pretty quick though, and I knew he was right—fruit juice *was* fruit juice, and exception number four was a bridge too far. I, being the rational, logical person that I am, dissolved into tears while accusing him of "not caring" about the project (*sniff*). I mean, I *wanted* those things, dammit! And shopping was suddenly and irrevocably getting, you know, *difficult*! I felt like Sisyphus rolling a giant powdered-sugar doughnut up a hill.

Secretly though, I *was* impressed: He cared! He was holding *me* to a higher standard! Wow. For the first time, I realized we really *were* in it all together...This crazy year would actually happen.

What had I done?

———

In the beginning, delivering us from temptation involved a three-pronged approach: unopened items with sugar went to the local food bank, opened items got eaten up (Quick! Eat this!) or thrown away, and items we couldn't possibly bear to part with (for example, the kids' Christmas candy) went into the freezer for the year.

———

I hate this project! I hate it! It's no fair. Mom is taking all the sweets in the house and giving them away. And she even is giving away our King Arthur Flour Kid's (baking) Kits: the Snickerdoodle and the Cowboy Chocolate Chipper Muffins. And she's giving away the

caramel popcorn that Grandpa just gave us a week or two
ago. I DON'T THINK IT'S FAIR!!

—*from Greta's journal*

Considering the rate at which I was getting rid of food at
our house, I needed to start replenishing in a big way. I made
plans for a trip to BJ's Wholesale Club. Because the closest BJ's is about an hour away from our house, getting there,
shopping, returning home, and unpacking usually takes the
better part of a day, so going there is kind of like an expe-
dition to Everest, with coupons. In the early weeks of the
project, I was fast learning to buy no-sugar items in quantity,
because we went through them quickly, and they could be
hard to find again. Consequently, I no longer bought one box
of no-sugar crackers; I bought four. I no longer bought one
jar of no-sugar peanut butter or tomato sauce; I bought six.
So a warehouse-store specializing in bulk was clearly a good
option—but BJ's only has what it has, so would I really find a
no-sugar version of everything I wanted?

Happily, I did manage to fill my cart, but not without
spending exactly *twice* as much time shopping as I used to,
and so much intense label reading that, rightfully, I should've
earned a degree of some kind. Over and over, I picked up
a package that listed sugar as the umpteenth ingredient
(gotcha!) only to go back to the drawing board and find
another brand of the same sort of item that (hooray!) did
not. Two seemingly identical bags of pistachios revealed their
true nature when flipped over: one had sugar listed among
three dozen other ingredients; the other listed pistachios and
sea salt.

See, now was that so hard? I thought. *Is it so hard to just put food in our food?*

Clearly, I was tired and cranky from all that small type, not to mention realizing that morning that I had to throw my favorite breakfast cereal out due to the presence of sugar. (Crispy Hexagons, how could you?) Sure, *some* sugar items are pretty blinking obvious—Nutella, hello?—but even a few weeks in, I continued to be blindsided by so many others, i.e., the number of "healthy" items that I was now forced to take an honest, unflinching look at. I began to think of it as the Evaporated Cane Syrup Brigade. *What? You mean I can't have Peanut Butter Clif Bars anymore? Wait, nobody told me that!*

Meanwhile, at dinner one night, Ilsa started describing the kind of little thingies-with-the-something-inside she would like for dessert, and I gently reminded her about the family project. She was sad for a moment but quickly rebounded, much to my surprise. Despite our preconceptions about the love affair between children and sugar, I started to wonder if the family project might actually end up being harder on Mom and Dad. After all, we had been around a lot longer; we'd had a lot longer to get hooked.

Nevertheless, I realized, it was time to start finding out if dessert was possible in a world of no sugar. We had given up sugar after all, not sweet. Ladies, start your Cuisinarts. The experiments were about to begin.

CHAPTER 5

EVERYTHING TASTES LIKE BANANAS AND DATES

Pretty soon, we found ourselves missing the myriad little things that sweeten up one's day—that little spark in your cereal, that spoonful of something in your afternoon tea, that bit of chocolate you might have after dinner for no particular reason. I couldn't shake that feeling after a meal that something was…missing. It was as if I'd just seen three quarters of a play when suddenly, the curtain goes down and everyone goes home. It had been so thoroughly ingrained in me to expect not only a sweet finale at the end of a meal but *especially* at the end of a labor-intensive home-cooked meal or a rare evening-out meal, that I found myself experiencing a sort of Phantom Dessert Syndrome. "What, no fireworks? No crème brûlée or tiramisu? Not so much as a *mint*?" my brain chemistry complained.

This deprived, waiting-for-the-other-shoe-to-drop feeling reminded me a lot of being pregnant. Both times I found out I was pregnant, I commenced the time-honored tradition of beginning to mildly lose my mind. Immediately, I swore off alcohol and caffeine. Also jaywalking, swimming within twenty-four hours of eating, and reading celebrity gossip.

Both times, it was the *beginning* that was hardest, trying to get used to the idea that something I regularly consumed and enjoyed was—whoops!—off the table. "Why, yes, I'd *love* a glass/cup of…of…I mean, uh, no. Thank you."

And as any woman who has ever been pregnant can tell you, one experiences hunger as if it is a brand-new sensation. After my fourteenth snack of the day, I'd go to bed and have vivid dreams about food in which I'm pretty sure I salivated and chewed in my sleep. Although I never dreamed I was eating a marshmallow and woke up to find my pillow gone, it was probably close.

I craved sweets, chocolate in particular. The catch was, every time I took a bite of anything chocolaty, the most peculiar thing happened: it would turn to dust in my mouth. Literally, it tasted as appetizing as wallpaper paste. So *other* desserts became, of course, quintessentially important.

Thus, one of my most memorable pregnant moments occurred at my cousin Gretchen's surprise fortieth birthday party for her husband. I was feeling large and uncomfortable, and the two-and-a-half-hour drive to get there seemed *much* longer. I recall floating my blimp-like self down to the ladies' room for what was my ninth or tenth visit when I was offered a beautiful slice of pastry—a Napoleon—by a passing waiter. Since I thought it perhaps in questionable taste to bring my dessert into the bathroom with me to pee, I demurred; I'd wait till I was back at my table.

Big mistake. *Huge.* By the time I returned to my table, there were *no* beautiful, fluffy, shiny little slices of Napoleon left. All gone. The alternative? Chocolate cake—for me, dust cake. Wallpaper-paste cake.

I sat in watery-eyed silence and longingly, resentfully

watched the guests at my table eat their desserts. *How* could *they?* I wondered with my pregnant-lady brain. I stopped just shy of sending my husband to announce from the balcony that there was a pregnant lady emergency and would some kind soul be willing to donate their Napoleon to a good cause?

I kid you not, I have *never* cared about a piece of food in my life as much as that untouchable Napoleon. So much of one's pregnancy is spent feeling hungry for some unnameable something that when you actually find the thing that will satisfy that hunger, it is as if the clouds have parted and the heavenly choir is singing. Then to have it snatched away? It was almost more than my hormone-addled brain could take. I was on the verge of tears in the car on the way home. I couldn't stop thinking about how deprived I felt, how I should've taken dessert with me to the bathroom, how unfair it was for everyone to have dessert but me. At that moment, it seemed as if there was a big hole in my middle that would remain hungry and incomplete—forever. All I can say is that those guests were lucky I wasn't armed.

Of course, looking back it all seems so ridiculous. Crying over a pastry? I have no idea what actual hunger really feels like, the kind that comes from genuine deprivation, and for that I am supremely grateful. At the risk of repeating myself, I know it's because our family is lucky enough to have enough food on a daily basis that we could make the privileged decision to carry out an experiment such as a sugarless year in the first place. Nobody in our family expects a medal for going without sugar cookies or chocolate bars for a year—but in this land of plenty, it is worth noting once again the amazing power food and our brain exert over us, expertly tricking us into thinking we *need* that chocolate bar, that can of pop, that Napoleon.

I'm here to tell you that despite everything my brain was telling me that day, I—and the baby in my belly that would one day be Greta—survived fine without it. And we would survive this year too—no violin music necessary, thank you.

That being said, no one in our family had interest in being masochistic for a year either. If we could find ways to fill that little empty spot in our gut, fool our brain chemistry into thinking we'd *had* a sugar treat, when in fact we had not, why not? More than that, it was a matter of family morale and my own personal sanity. The kids didn't want to hear me paraphrasing comic book philosophy: "with great food variety comes great responsibility."[22] They wanted what every American kid wants: Popsicles. Cookies. Ice cream.

Lucky for us, we had inherited from Steve's father both a Champion juicer machine *and* the World's Shortest Ice Cream Recipe, which not only contains no added sugar, but also contains only one ingredient: bananas. So here it is: peel bananas, freeze on a cookie sheet, run them through the juicer. Voilà! Soft-serve banana ice cream!

———————

...we had dessert a couple nights ago. Maybe I'd better explain. We had homemade banana ice cream. Homemade ice cream you can make without sugar. Or some people might call it cold puree. But I say, if I might have a say, I think it's ice cream. All it is, is frozen bananas put

———————————————————————

[22]Get it? "With great power comes great responsibility"? Spiderman's Uncle Ben? Oh, never mind.

in a machine and out it comes—no sugar. So we aren't
naughty. Yet.

—from Greta's journal

In the early days of our Year of No Sugar, Bill Schaub's banana ice cream became our go-to lifesaver-recipe; we had it at least once a week. Its only drawback being—like so many things we would cook, make, and bake in our year—it takes *time*. One night we were SO proud and excited about our first No Sugar dessert that we tried to make it spontaneously for a friend and her kids. The consequence of not quite enough freezer time, however, ended up being that our dessert was more akin to banana *pudding* than ice cream…still, our family all ate our bowls up with vigor. Our friend and her kids, however—who apparently weren't as sugar-starved as we were—seemed less than impressed.

Still. If we were going to last a whole year without *going* bananas, we needed more than just one dessert. Clearly, the time had come to improvise. There was only one problem. I've never been very good at improvising. I am, I'm afraid, heartbreakingly literal in some ways—*especially* when it comes to food.

Just ask Katrina. She's the friend who made me realize it was perhaps—just *perhaps*—a teensy bit *rigid* to time the macaroni cooking to the second, just to make a box of Annie's Mac & Cheese (in point of fact, she burst out laughing). Have I made this mom-staple three thousand times? Yes. No matter. It took an extreme force of will to get me to dump the pasta out a few seconds early, and it would plainly never have occurred to me to dump the milk in *unmeasured*. Gasp!

In fact, up until this particular year, I had been known not to make a recipe at all for lack of a single, tangential ingredient, such as half a teaspoon of tarragon. After all, I reasoned, that might *make* the dish! And why go through all the effort to make something not as good as it is supposed to be? (Perhaps this was residual blowback from that far-off mud cake I had made as a kid without that half-teaspoon of baking powder.)

But on the No-Sugar Project, my improvising wings were forced to take flight, for better or worse. It started with me bravely leaving out a teaspoon of table sugar here, a tablespoon of honey there. And so far everything had been fine! Really! *Surprisingly* so. I baked baguettes *without* three-fourths of a teaspoon of sugar, cheddar cheese soup *without* Worcestershire sauce (couldn't find a no-sugar version), and sweet potato biscuits *without* two tablespoons sugar. I was on a roll.

So I tried making an apricot bar recipe that we had loved in the past, but omitting the three-quarters of a cup of brown sugar called for in the butter and flour crust. Now three-quarters of a cup is a *lot* more than a tablespoon, and I realized some sort of replacement would be necessary to round out the crust and provide it with the correct density and stick-together-y-ness. I ended up trying three-quarters of a cup mushed banana. I felt very adventurous and confident we'd end up with an inedible mess.

Yet, amazingly, the apricot bars were not just edible; they were actually *good*! Turns out, the banana pulp provided just the right amount of stickiness to form a proper crust and emitted a delicious, sweet smell while baking. Of course, the bars weren't nearly as sweet as before, but they *were* sweet, primarily due to the cooked apricot filling. They failed to brown nicely on the top, but this problem was solved down the road with the addition of egg to the crust ingredients.

So far, I had yet to hack any failed experiments into the trash with an ice pick. I was astounded. Perhaps there was something *to* this winging-it approach.

I found other recipes online and continued experimenting; there was a nice raisin and apple cookie that could be a little awkwardly concocted by sautéing the fruit then adding it to the dry ingredients, and chilling it in the fridge overnight before baking. After weeks of thinking wistfully of treats gone by, I was ecstatic to simply *eat a cookie* again, although I secretly worried some aspect of the "banana pudding effect" might still be at work, to wit: it only tastes good to us because we were—to put it nicely—desperate.

No matter. I was coming to realize that treats are in the eye of the beholder. Emboldened by my first few attempts, I began altering cookie recipes that had been long-held favorites in our house: peanut butter, oatmeal raisin, Nestle Toll House chocolate chip. I tried to develop a system of sorts, a kind of No-Sugar Conversion Chart: in place of white sugar, I would use an equivalent amount of mashed banana; in place of brown sugar, that amount of chopped dates; and in place of chocolate chips, carob chips. (It wouldn't be until much later in the year that I would realize carob too was, in fact, off the table for us, being a processed sweetener itself. It would not be our first mistake, and certainly was not our last.) These experiments were simultaneously heartening and disappointing. On the one hand, they all resulted in solid, reliable, sweet, no-sugar cookies. I brought them to knitting night and potlucks, offered them to our friend's children. Even the non-sugar-starved agreed—they were pretty good cookies.

Not "the-best-cookie-you-ever-ate" good, but good enough that every kid I gave them to said "yummy" and ate the whole thing. (I feel kids are the most dependable taste testers because they're the ones who have no qualms about spitting a cookie out on your linoleum, whether it hurts your feelings or not.) The big problem with my No-Sugar Conversion Chart, however, was this: everything came out *the same*—tasting like bananas and dates. The peanut butter cookies tasted like bananas and dates. The oatmeal raisin and the carob chip? Like bananas and dates. Sure, they were serviceable recipes, but due to the fact that my sweetening agents had some rather loud tastes of their own to express (BANANA! DATE!), they only really made *one* cookie.

Nevertheless it was really, *really* nice to be able to put a cookie in each of our kid's lunches in the morning; like so many times in the past when I had sent sugar desserts, I felt like I was sending them a little edible love note. I realized sugar wasn't the only thing I felt starved of—it was also the very concept of being able to provide a treat as a sign of affection. After all, if sugar is used as a symbol of affection (which it surely is—just ask the people who sell heart-shaped boxes of candy), then what does that make the lady who imposes on her family a Year of No Sugar? The Anti-Mommy? The culinary equivalent of Joan Crawford? The Grinch?

As if this weren't bad enough, in abstaining from sugar, we were, naturally, going to have to stay away from one of the key "crops" of our many neighbors: maple syrup. We live in Vermont, after all, famous to the world for pretty much three things: fall foliage, straight-shooting but excitable presidential candidates, and maple syrup. Thus, not only were we abandoning *love* in the form of sugar, we were also abandoning some very real component of local pride or patriotism that took the form of sugar.

If you don't live here, I think it's hard to fully appreciate the impact that maple syrup, and its related products—maple ("Indian") sugar, maple sugar candy, maple cream, maple creemies (soft-serve ice cream), maple cotton candy, maple roasted nuts, and so on—have on the culture, economy, and collective unconscious of Vermont. Just look at our state quarter: a guy straight out of Vermont-stereotype casting, sporting a plaid jacket and sugaring with buckets the old-fashioned way. (Although metal sap buckets are still used here and there, the preferred modern method involves a much less bucolic plastic sap line, which runs from tree to tree. Come springtime, you'll see them materialize on trees like quick-climbing vines.)

Now here is some surprising advice, coming from me: if you've never had maple syrup fresh, by which I mean straight out of the boiling-down process, this is an experience you must try to have in your lifetime, because there is no other taste in the world like it. Unless you are attempting your own Year of No Sugar, I see no real obstacles for you, save getting through the almost-as-famous Vermont mud in springtime. There is some sort of magic that is happening just then, as the water is evaporated out of the sap slowly, hovered over for hours in the warmth of the sugarhouse, that you can actually taste at no other time than right then. Likely, you will have wind-burned cheeks and be stamping your slushy shoes when someone hands you a Dixie cup containing a tablespoon or two of warm, pure gold. Warning: your taste buds may very well be spoiled forever.

You may never even want to have regular maple syrup

again. All things considered, having one tablespoon of that just-born manna might be a great trade-off for all those metal gallons we might otherwise go through. In fact (and I'm going to speak *very* quietly now, so my fellow Vermonters won't hear me), after Steve devised a new-and-improved pancake recipe employing coconut and (what else?) bananas, we found we could enjoy no-syrup pancakes very well, and without that "maple-syrup crash" half an hour later.

It's tough though. I'm a stickler for appreciating culture, heritage, history. Of all the sugars on our list, maple sugar might well be the most appealing from a romantic and historical point of view. It's hard to be nostalgic about sugar extracted by machines from beets or corn. But extracting maple sap from the shady trees that dot our state is something almost anyone can do with a proper hammer and tin bucket. This appeals, of course, not only to history buffs who see continuity stretching back even to the Native Americans, but also to the do-it-yourself mentality that is so entrenched throughout New England.

We know people who sugar every year for fun, and those who do so for serious profit. We know people with sleek, modern sap boilers and those whose impossible, heaving contraptions look as if they belong in the Middle Ages. We have sat in on lengthy discussions of wood fire versus propane heating and whether or not you can properly cook a batch down on your stove without ending up with a flypaper-wall kitchen and whether you can taste the difference when some of the trees happen to grow just over the line in (gasp!) New York. We know people who use no sweetener besides maple syrup—in their coffee, their baking, in their glazed carrots and sweet potatoes.

Believe me when I say, maple syrup is waaaaaaay beyond a thing to put on your pancakes around here. It's practically a religion.

Which makes me...? Once again, the bad guy? If this were *Star Wars*, would I be the creepy old guy in the black hood in desperate need of a facial and some eye drops?

No. I was determined. I was *not* going to be the Sugar Nazi; I was not—probably—going to instill neurosis in my children that would haunt them for decades to come. I believed, with perhaps Pollyanna-ish determination, that we should be able to eat *without* sugar *without* being miserable.

Which is *not* to say without pissing anybody off.

CHAPTER 6

WAITRESSES HATE US

It didn't take long for me to become familiar with "The Look." "The Look" is that mixture of dismay and confusion which appears on the waiter, cashier, or cafeteria line lady's face when asked if the penne with red peppers and broccoli has sugar in it.

"*Sugar* in it?" they always said, as if they perhaps didn't hear me correctly.

Sigh.

The thing is, I'm really not cut out for this sort of thing at all. If I were, I would be reveling in the chance to tell our story to each and every new waitress, enlightening her with The Truth About Fructose as if I had discovered it hovering above a burning bush. I would keenly expound on a handful of salient facts and shocking statistics, captivating her for just enough time to pique her interest and handing her my card at just the right moment, along with another one for the chef in the back.

The only problem being, I suck at this. If eloquent, persuasive speech were like dancing, I'd be Jerry Lewis on stage during *Swan Lake*.

My husband, on the other hand, is amazing at this sort of thing. You've heard of the guy who can sell snow to Eskimos? Water to fish? Redneck jokes to Jeff Foxworthy? That's my husband. Everywhere we go *he's* the one who's telling people just the right amount of information about our Year of No Sugar. And complete strangers lean over and listen, captivated.

But me? Nope. And it's not just with waitstaff and counter people, but friends, relatives, acquaintances; I can pinpoint almost the exact moment when the other person's face changes. If there were words running across their forehead like a stock ticker they would read: "*Uh*-oh. Here it comes." It's that moment when I start telling them about the No-Sugar Project.

So when I'm at a bonfire party, say, and my daughter runs up to me, complaining about the fact that there isn't anything to drink but apple cider and what should she *do*, then, turning back to the curious person I was talking to, I go into Explaining Mode. Half apologetic, I relate the *Reader's Digest* version of our Family Project, carefully monitoring the listener's face for the telltale switch from curiosity to boredom, repulsion, defensiveness.

Of course, most friends and acquaintances are way too gracious to express these negative reactions outright, so instead I get the forehead ticker. Something ever-so-subtle shifts in their posture toward me, and they assume the expression of someone who is politely interested yet has no intention of changing any aspect of their current life, thank you very much. They are ever so subtly on their guard, as if I had casually turned the conversation toward the fact that aliens talk to me through my toaster oven.

In such a conversation, I can't help but feel anxious that

the other person will feel put-upon, like I'm trying to tell them **What To Do**—like I'm sooooooo smart that I have all the answers. I never feel that way. I never have all the answers. A motivational speaker I will never be.

Which is probably why I'm a writer and not on TV selling Sham Wows. It's also probably why I spent the year being pretty sure waitresses hated us. It was not unusual, for example, for our questions about the *this*, the *that*, and the *the other* to send the waitress scurrying back to the kitchen three or four times before we could arrive at an actual meal order. If you were a waitress, wouldn't *you* hate us?

Yet I can honestly report with amazement that we never encountered actual, definable rudeness regarding our project from any source. No one ever told us it was stupid, for example, or encouraged us to flake off. Rather, it was more on the order of piling inconvenience on top of inconvenience. For example, when we ate at the new Thai restaurant on a busy evening, the response to whether the pad thai contained any sugar or not was followed by our waiter abandoning us for twenty minutes. By the time he returned, we were all hungry enough to eat our laminated menus. When the answer turned out to be yes, the pad thai contains sugar, we asked about another dish and he disappeared again. Meanwhile, other tables were having drinks, receiving plates of food, even people who had come in long after we had arrived were *eating actual food* while we had yet to decide on an order. When he finally returned again, Steve gave me a grim look that wordlessly said "DO NOT, UNDER ANY CIRCUMSTANCES, ASK ANY MORE QUESTIONS." In desperation, I guessed at an innocuous-sounding noodle dish that I later concluded most assuredly had honey in it. Sigh.

On the other hand, some places were astoundingly accommodating, which is still not to say easy. For example, in March for two weeks, I accompanied my father to the Mayo Clinic—a world-renowned medical facility in Rochester, Minnesota. We were investigating some longstanding and worsening medical problems that had been confounding his doctors back home, and it was time for the experts to be superseded by *the experts*.

The Mayo Clinic, by definition, is an extremely humbling place. Although certainly this is not true of everyone, many of the people who are there are there as an extreme, if not last, medical resort. Of course, you never know *why* someone is at Mayo, or even which person in a group of people might be the patient, but wandering around, you do tend to look at folks and wonder, *Why is* she *here? Is it* him? All these people are suffering in some way, some more obviously than others.

Occasionally I would notice someone red-eyed and sniffling into a Kleenex as we sat down in one of the many waiting rooms. What could anyone really say? Or do? Who knows what news they may have just received? And then you see *children* with parents heading to an appointment and you just pray they are here for something ridiculously benign, like an inverted hangnail.

One day, I met a woman at the hotel's laundry machines who explained without prompting that her husband was so ill—with pancreatitis, I think it was—that she couldn't leave him in the room alone very long. As we were talking, she got a cell phone call to tell her that, by the way, her nephew had been diagnosed with cancer.

Suffice it to say, it's a heck of a perspective check, on top of which was the fact that I was pretty darned worried about my dad. In the face of obvious suffering and illness of every variety, it was certainly tempting to feel like our family's little project was so...so...self-centered. Irrelevant. Egotistical even. *Why* was I torturing our family again, anyway? *Who* cared what we had to eat every day?

And yet, one day, as I sat idly waiting for my dad in the clinic coffee shop, I was bemused and then, gradually, alarmed to observe how many people came in to grab a soda. Pepsi. Pepsi. Diet Coke. Sprite. Coke. Hardly a minute went by without a hand opening the soda cooler across from me—and *no one*, I realized, was taking water. Once again, I had that weird sensation of being the only person in the room who could see a possible connection between rampant sugar and rampant suffering.

Then later, I passed by the Mayo "Center for Tobacco-Free Living" and I wondered: would there ever be a Mayo "Center for Sugar-Free Living"? Who knows how many people at Mayo at that very moment suffered from metabolic syndrome? Who knows how many might have been helped by the knowledge contained in that YouTube video I had watched what now seemed like so long ago? *I* wasn't going to provide any answers—not honest-to-goodness, double-blind, proven medical ones—but I really did believe it was time to at least *begin this conversation*. Which was, in fact, what I was trying to do, in my own weird little way.

Lucky for me, I probably couldn't have found any place on earth as willing to accommodate my ingredient queries as they were there. Because of the clinic—which in employing some 33,000 people, coupled with accommodating some 350,000 patients every year essentially *is* the town of

Rochester—they are used to fielding just about every kind of question you can ask about food. *So* many folks there have restrictions, special diets, or upcoming test requirements that the waitstaff are experts on things most restaurant staff haven't the vaguest idea about. But even the diabetics weren't asking *quite* the same question that I was asking. Usually, I would preface it by saying, "I have a little bit of a weird question…"

Also very helpful was the box of Kashi cereal I had packed in my suitcase. One of the surprising things I learned during our Year of No Sugar is the fact that the hardest meal of the day is *breakfast*…hands down. Just take a look at it and you'll see what I mean: there's cereal (added sugar), toast or bagels (added sugar), juice (*is* sugar), waffles (added sugar, and that's even before the syrup), muffins and Danishes (oh, come *on!*)…Pretty much black coffee and eggs *without* toast and *without* bacon are what you are left with. Ew.

I feel more and more ambivalent about this project every day. It's just so confusing. I mean, me and my family can only eat four kinds of cereal now. Well, it's not like it's a big drop, but it's something. That means, like, we never ate Cocoa Puffs, Lucky Charms, or Fruit Loops. We ate stuff like Crispy Hexagons and Gorilla Munch. Now we can only have 7 Whole Grain Puffs, Shredded Wheat (shaped like big hay bales), the small shredded wheat original, and 7 Whole Grain Nuggets—Boring. But then there's the other agenda. Mom can still make oatmeal, just can't put maple syrup on it. Also, Mom leaves out the sugar in the pancakes and puts blueberries in to sweeten it. We had pancakes this morning and, boy, were they good!! Even if we can't put on maple syrup.

So as you can see here today, I wrote about the breakfast situation.

See you—Greta
—from Greta's journal

I stealthily smuggled my cereal into the complimentary hotel breakfast bar each morning, brazenly making use of their Styrofoam bowls, plastic spoons, and paper napkins, as well as a heap of raisins, which had been originally betrothed to some instant, sugar-containing oatmeal, before being abducted and eloping with my 7 Whole Grain Nuggets at the last minute. It seemed a pretty good solution until we had been there for over a week, and I began to feel that if I ate any more whole grain nuggets I would jump off the nearest whole grain ledge.

Harder still were the weekends. Why? Because on Saturdays and Sundays, the Mayo Clinic is closed and, consequently, so are a *whole* lot of the restaurants. What stays open is just the kind of food I totally couldn't eat: sub chains and coffee shops. In the sub shop, the meats are usually cooked with glazes and other additives that are likely to include sugar, and the bread usually has it too; coffee shops are basically one big dessert.

So, having little other choice, on Saturday night, I took my dad to the sub chain inside our hotel. While he ordered his sandwich I noticed that they had a "no carb" option of wrapping your ingredients inside a large lettuce leaf rather than their bread (which—I checked—had sugar). Rather than enter into a ten-hour discussion of the ingredients of the various cold cuts, I ordered the veggie sub *with* the no-carb option—basically a vegetable bonanza, with a slice of cheese thrown in there for good measure. I couldn't very well add mayonnaise because *that* has sugar (oh yes!) so I slathered on some mustard and dug into a *very* crunchy meal. Food? Yes. Satisfying? Decidedly not.

The next day was equally tricky. After a good breakfast of plain oatmeal and berries at a nearby hotel, I thought I was probably full enough to get through till an early dinner. Not so much. I really should realize this about my metabolism by now, but somehow I still regularly manage to convince myself that maybe I don't *really* need to eat all three meals if it isn't entirely convenient. In fact, I am like a wind-up toy that stops working when its short little energy supply runs out.

So there I was, sitting in my beige hotel room, midafternoon, dinner still *hours* away, and not a thing in sight to eat. As usual when I miss a meal, I began to feel slightly ill—and then desperate. The Larabar from my suitcase (ingredients: nuts, whole dried fruit) had helped, but not enough. I couldn't face another vegetable sandwich wrapped in lettuce…but then I had an idea. I went to the counter at the sub shop and asked if I could just order some cheese.

"Just *cheese*?" the scruffy, twentysomething man behind the counter asked, blinking. He checked with the sandwich makers behind him. "We can do *just* cheese, right?"

No one could think of any reason not to sell me some cheese. "Hey, there's no reason why we can't!" he said brightly, and he rang it up. The cheese came to seventy-five cents.

After checking the ingredients, I also added a bag of potato chips and received my tiny little package of cheese from the pick-up counter.

Back in my room, I was sorry to see they had only given me two small pieces. I should've asked for two or three servings' worth. Oh well—paired with the banana I had stolen from the largely inedible (for me) breakfast bar and the chips, it still made a serviceable lunch.

It was all there: I had some carbohydrates, some salt, some fat, and some fructose wrapped—as it should be—in its corresponding fiber and micronutrients. I was happy with my little improvised meal and even happier that it put a stop to the gnawing in my belly.

And honestly, it was waaaaay better than a lettuce and mustard sandwich.

In our entire year, in fact, there was only one time that I felt too intimidated to even *ask* about the sugar content of the menu items. It was over the kids' February break. We had decided to make a trip to Philadelphia and see some fun historic sites: Independence Hall, the Liberty Bell, Ben Franklin's outhouse—the works.

Evidently our hotel had never heard of the "complimentary breakfast" phenomenon that is sweeping the rest of the Western world, so we ate almost every day at a small diner around the corner. It was the kind of place that's so retro they don't even *know* they're retro. I was in love with the Formica U-shaped counters lined with swiveling chrome stools.

Now, I'm not sure if it was the Russian waitress with three stars tattooed behind her right ear, the two local guys who came in every morning and ordered Coke with their French toast, or the fact that there would simply be nothing left for us to eat but eggs with eggs and eggs on the side, but I just *couldn't* bring myself to ask. I just couldn't.

So, primarily, we stuck to the things we *knew* were safe: bland, unsweetened oatmeal; grapefruit; and of course, eggs. But we were still *hungry*.

In desperation, I enacted the "Philadelphia Breakfast Exemption," which read as follows: *Don't* ask about the bread. Just don't.

After we had democratically seconded the motion and passed the emergency measure by a clear margin, we gratefully enjoyed some whole-wheat toast and bagels during our stay. Was there a really, really good chance there was *some* amount of sugar in those bread products? Like a thirty-second of a teaspoon? Yes. I was determined, however, not to let such an emergency situation happen again.

Consequently I now present to you, dear reader, the Official Waitress Interrogating Primer: or How to Make Sure Your Food is Free of Fructose, If Not Waitress Spit:

1. Have your meal at an "off" time to ensure you can take a few minutes for questions without pissing off the entire restaurant. Early is better than later, of course, since by 9 p.m. your waiter/waitress may be out of patience for the evening.

2. I prefer to let the waitperson settle us in and get us drinks ("Girls, would you like water or milk?") before attacking her with our concerns. When, in the absence of milk, the waitperson helpfully offers the kids Yoo-hoo ("Girls, would you like water or partially hydrogenated soybean oil?"), politely wave off the suggestion and order them water.

3. When drinks are brought back, broach the subject. I like to say, "I'm sorry, but sugar in any form makes me immediately and violently ill. Can you recommend a menu item that wouldn't involve me frightening your other customers?" Or, "Ever since we came to the realization that sugar is the devil's food, we've been abstaining from it. Would you like to read some complimentary literature we have on the subject?"

Okay, actually, what I *really* say is this, verbatim, every time: "I have a bit of a strange question. We're not eating (ever-so-subtle pause, followed by delicate emphasis)...Any. Added. Sugar. (Follow-up pause.) I was looking at the sautéed beef tongue, but I was concerned about...*the sauce*. Do you think you could check with the kitchen for me on that?" And then—and this is key—BEFORE your waiter disappears in the great maw of the kitchen, never to return again, quickly ask about *any other items your family is considering ordering*. Although he/she might be temporarily annoyed at having to deviate from the ordinary waiter-client script, believe me, he/she will appreciate not having to make seven separate trips to interrogate the chef—and you won't have to have your dinner at one in the morning, while the cleanup crew vacuums ever-so-subtly under your feet.

4. ALWAYS be excessively grateful for the extra time your waitperson has dedicated to your crazy-ass requests. "Thank you *again* for your help," goes a long way if you ever want to return to this establishment, and so does a generous tip, which I highly recommend unless they pulled the Disappearing Waitstaff Trick on you.

In our year, we found it helpful, and a relief, to get to know the menus of the restaurants in our area and which items on the menu we could have without fear of sugar sneaking. We were lucky to find one (!!) wonderful, reasonably priced bistro nearby that made nearly everything from scratch and whose waitresses became so used to our requests that they'd know what we wanted before we ordered it—and who regularly asked us how the No-Sugar Thing was going. The kind of place where the specials are written in colorful marker on a piece of cardstock. The kind of place where they put homemade French bread pizza on the children's menu simply because Ilsa requested it so often. This familiar establishment practically brought tears of gratitude to my eyes at the end of a week of cooking sauces, breads, and chicken broth from scratch. All I can say is—thank God for The Trolley Stop.

In Poultney, Vermont.

Please tell them I sent you.

Of course, you're going to have to keep in mind that you're not going to be eating at any fast food or all-you-can-eat *anything*. Generally speaking, the restaurants will have to be sit-down and of the variety that makes at least some portion of their food from scratch. Once you start to ask, you'll be amazed at the number of restaurants in which the ingredients are an absolute mystery to everyone—including the "chef" (we are using the term loosely here). How can this be? Because the food arrives at the establishment *already made*— sauces, pastas, meat dishes—and all your restaurant does is heat them up. Ma's Kountry Cookin' indeed.

After a while, you will come to learn that there is always, *always* sugar in the sauce. Also, the dressing, the breading, and very, *very* likely the soup. Remember: even *ingredients* have ingredients. Chicken broth *sounds* fine, right? But unless it's made in house, I will bet you my sweet Aunt Matilda it has added sugar. When dining in restaurants, the safest bets are always the plainest ones: steak with fries. Fish with vegetables. Spaghetti with garlic and oil. While traveling in Minnesota with my dad, I had a staggering amount of baked walleye with steamed vegetables—yum! (And I had never even *heard* of walleye before. See the new worlds No Sugar can open up to you?)

After a while, you too will come to know in advance which items are Generally Pretty Safe. Ironically, we sometimes found ourselves in the position of having to choose the French fries or the potato chips over the whole-grain bread basket— but such was the nature of our challenge. If we hadn't realized it before, we were certainly becoming acquainted with it now: not eating added sugar as a family was a gargantuan endeavor. No one ever said everything we ate was going to be healthy on every *other* account.

CHAPTER 7

OH, THE THINGS YOU WILL EAT

You'd think it'd be simple to exclude sugar from your diet, right? Not *easy* perhaps, but at least reasonably *simple*. You wouldn't have to be Einstein. Just look at the ingredients, and then when you find sugar—*don't eat it*. Right? Simple. Yet right away, we began running into mysterious ingredients that seemed bent on defying my foolproof plan.

"But *what about...?*" became our constant refrain. Like a Whac-A-Mole game gone wrong, just as we painstakingly resolved one "can we or can't we?" issue, another would pop up to take its place. In our Year of No Sugar, we needed a litmus test.

This brings us to the part that trips a lot of folks up. I wish I had a dime for every time someone has said to me, "But WAIT! If you're *just* avoiding fructose/still eating fruit/ still eating pasta, you're *still eating sugar*, right?" Well, that depends on what you mean by "sugar." Remember, *table* sugar (aka sucrose) is made up of roughly equal parts glucose and fructose; glucose is what your body wants. It is the gas that makes the car (your body) go. Some foods convert quite readily to glucose (breads, pastas, and other simple carbohydrates, for example) while others require more work and time to convert (meats and other proteins). This is why diabetics have to watch not just what they eat, but also in what proportion they eat it—too many slices of bread can send their blood sugar skyrocketing.

So, were we talking about a year of no *blood* sugar? Which is to say a year of no *glucose*? Well, no, not unless we were trying to starve ourselves to death.

When we said a Year of No Sugar, we meant a Year of No Added Fructose. Why are these two terms equivalent? Because you can have sugar without glucose and you can have glucose without sugar, *but you can't have sugar without fructose and you can't have fructose without sugar*. Fructose is what makes sugar, sugar. And at the risk of beating this dead horse into dust particles: fructose *is the bad guy*; if our diet were a western film, fructose would be wearing the black hat and spitting chewing tobacco at children and small animals. Fructose, you'll recall, is poison. Fructose is the ingredient that our body can live entirely without, thank you very much, and would be much the better off for it.

But because fructose is so *delicious*, and perhaps even *addictive*, we brilliant humans have farmed fructose, extracted fructose, injected fructose into every darned thing we can get our hands on—from bacon to baby formula. Actual fruit, which is where fructose naturally comes from, contains comparatively small amounts of fructose and so is the least of our worries. The problem is not the fruit—whose fiber and micronutrients make up for the tiny bit of fructose-poison that goes along for the ride—the problem is *every-bloody-thing else*. The problem, in a nutshell, is *added* fructose—in short, nature got it right

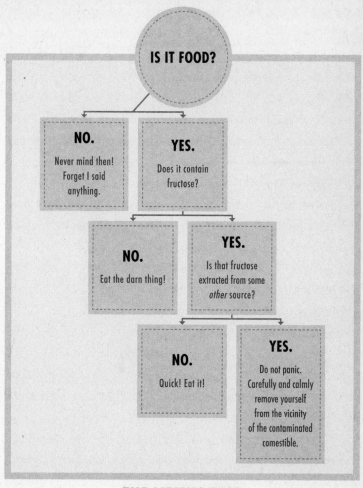

THE LITMUS TEST

and know-it-all-humans continue to get it horribly wrong. This is why *apples* are good but apple *juice* is bad.[23] And if you

---

[23]How many times have I looked over in a restaurant to see a child enjoying French toast and apple juice and wondered if the parents would be equally fine with ordering them the nutritional equivalents of cake and soda for breakfast instead?

start to look, you will realize that added fructose, under all its guises and pen names, is in virtually every single package of food that you can buy.

So whenever someone asked me, as they inevitably would, "Oh, you're *only* avoiding *fructose?*" as if our family were swearing off avocados or pâté for the year, instead of the whole damn supermarket, you'll forgive me if I tended to get a little exasperated.

Back to the litmus test. Because the Dr. Lustig–inspired line of reasoning held that fructose was nutritional evil, whenever evaluating some murky or questionable ingredient, I always looked to three questions:

Is it food?

Does it contain fructose? And,

Is that fructose extracted from some other source?

Some questions were easy. Take medicine. As the song goes: "A spoonful of sugar makes the medicine go down..." Although, to be more accurate, we could say a spoonful of high-fructose corn syrup, sucralose, and Red Dye #40 makes the medicine go down.

Now, as an obsessive and overprotective mom, medicine was *off* the table as far as I was concerned. *Way* off. It wasn't even in the same *room* as the table. No-Sugar Project or no, if my child was sick, I was not, repeat, *not* going to quibble about trying to find no-sugar Children's Tylenol or some effective alternative to a tablespoon of canned fruit syrup to quiet a seriously upset tummy. (Did you know about that one? It works.) Nope. Medicine is *not food*; it's a whole other category.

That being said, using my new superpower of heightened sugar awareness, I was nonetheless a little horrified to note that the drug industry has clearly gotten on board the "more is more" wagon when it came to adding sugar to their products. This is definitely recent. Do you remember the days when taking medicine—*any* kind of medicine—was just *awful?* Like, gag-reflex-inducing awful? I'm not saying we should bring back the bad ol' days when we had to compound *feeling* like crap with taking medicine which *tasted* like crap, but it is troubling to notice that standard medicine cabinet items, such as fever reducer and cough drops, have been essentially transformed into *candy*. Ask any mom: it's to the point where kids beg to have additional unnecessary doses. Now that kind of scares me.

Nonetheless, the question of medicine was easily dispatched with. But here came the Whac-A-Mole—what about *vitamins?* A friend pointed out to me that the children's chewable vitamins prescribed by our pediatrician almost certainly have sugar in them to make them palatable. This was a tougher question. Vitamins aren't quite medicine, yet neither are they food. After some thought, I decided that since they are an item we get by prescription (no Flintstone Gummies here), they would remain in the medicine category, and therefore be permissible.[24]

Then came another tricky one. One day it came to my attention that although we weren't drinking fruit juice or consuming anything sweetened *with* fruit juice, there was nevertheless one fruit juice we still were consuming: lemon juice. As my home cooking had stepped up to fill the void of packaged and boxed foods in our lives, I found I was relying on the tartness of lemon quite a bit: in my homemade salad

---

[24]Thanks to a new label I have recently discovered, our kids' prescription vitamins, in fact, do not contain added sugar. Yay!

dressing, my homemade hummus, and several different pasta and vegetable recipes. But because I wasn't using it for *sweetening*, it didn't immediately register with me that it *was*, of course, still fruit juice. Could I somehow justify lemon juice on the No-Sugar Project?

So, I did some research. According to the handy-dandy nutrient calculator found on the USDA National Nutrient Database[25] there are <u>0.53 grams</u> of fructose in the 48 grams of juice in an average lemon. So if we compare apples to apples, so to speak, how does it measure up? If I was using the nutrient calculator correctly—of which there is absolutely no guarantee—48 grams of unsweetened apple juice comes in at 2.75 grams of fructose, so about *five times* as much fructose as in lemon juice. And 48 grams is about *one-fourth of a cup* of apple juice, not a drinking glass full.[26]

After much soul searching, I decided that a tablespoon of lemon juice, which was not sweet and carried a fraction of the fructose load of other common fruits, would be allowed here and there. So shoot me.

And then there were beverages. Now, do you *know* how many drinks are verboten on No Added Sugar? *All* of them. Okay, I exaggerate. *Most* of them. Virtually the entire drink menu/beverage aisle/vending machine lineup everywhere you go contains ample fructose: obviously soda and juice, but also anything even remotely interesting—from lemonade and

---

[25]United States Department of Agriculture, National Nutrient Database for Standard Reference http://ndb.nal.usda.gov/ndb/foods/show/2274?fg=&man=&lfacet=&count=&max=25&sort=&qlookup=lemon&offset=&format=Full&new=

[26]An eight-ounce glass of juice might be considered standard. How much fructose would be in *that*? Approximately 12.99 grams.

iced teas to hot cocoa, apple cider, flavored milks, and vitamin waters. Of course, we don't *need* anything other than water, right? Right?

But for our purposes, we did have a *small* range of choice. In addition to good old regular water, we had sparkling water (fancy!) and milk, as well as unsweetened coffee or tea for the grown-ups. Maybe it's telling that both Steve's and my one-item exceptions for the year (his: diet soda, mine: wine) were both beverages. Our society just loooooves to improve on water. However, because we were accustomed to a land of limitless choices (if sugar in a variety of textures, colors, and artificial flavorings *is* choice), in the interest of family morale, I was constantly on the lookout for any form of beverage variety we could find.

Then one day I came across a throwback beverage: Ovaltine. And before you can say "*Ovaltine?*" I must clarify that this was not the very same Ovaltine for which so many adult Americans are nostalgic and with whose labels one might have once sent away for a Little Orphan Annie decoder ring. In *that* Ovaltine, sugar is the number one ingredient. No, this was *European* Ovaltine that I came across at the famous Vermont Country Store, which prides itself on purveying hard-to-find items that are nonetheless still beloved by *somebody* out there—such as "Gee Your Hair Smells Terrific" shampoo, "Tigress" perfume ("Are you wild enough to wear it?"), and, my personal favorite, cod liver oil. Yup. Just in case anybody out there was feeling nostalgic about *that* stuff.

Presumably Europeans are fussier than Americans about how they like their hot beverages and, as with tea or coffee, prefer to add the amount of sugar that suits their specific taste. Finding this product made my month. Adding it to warm milk created a hot chocolate-ish experience[27] without the sugar, and we all immediately commenced enjoying it for breakfast and snacks.

Not long after that, I encountered another candidate for our oh-so-selective Club of Beverages. I picked up a bottle from the case of our local health store with curiosity. Hmmmmm, what *is* "coconut water"? I wondered. Did it count as fruit juice or something else? Again, some sleuthing was in order.

As it turned out, coconut water was no European Ovaltine, or even lemon juice for that matter. According to Livestrong.com, a serving of coconut water has 5.4 grams of combined simple sugars: glucose and fructose. No matter how you sliced it, that *had* to be quite a bit of fructose—similar to the amount found in apple juice. Too bad. Coconut water was out.

———

Of course, we were enjoying fruits of all shapes and sizes, and I had had a degree of success with my banana-, date-, and coconut-sweetened baked goods. But I wanted more. My tummy was crying out for something satisfying that didn't taste like it was plucked from Carmen Miranda's hat.

For the most part, the alternative sweeteners you'll find used as ingredients in the products on the shelves of the health food store or in the health food aisle at the supermarket are

---

[27]European Ovaltine's ingredients are things like malt extract, milk, cocoa powder, whey, and a slew of elaborate-sounding vitamins (such as "ferric orthophosphate" and "thiamine mononitrate"). Not exactly Michael Pollan's five ingredients or fewer, but we'd take it.

pretty disappointing. "Evaporated cane syrup" and "organic apple juice" *sound* a lot healthier and nicer, but in fact aren't any better fructose-wise than their high-fructose corn syrup counterparts (and in some cases they're worse—more on that in a minute).

Now some people think sugar is simply sugar. But that unfortunately isn't the case. To trick the shoppers into thinking there isn't sugar, they put in other things. But there is also simply sugar in different forms. Like evaporated cane juice—that's sugar. It's only a matter of being raw and evaporated. Also…high-fructose corn syrup. A last two are molasses and also fruit juice.

—from Greta's journal

"Barley malt syrup" cropped up in ingredient lists occasionally, which was something we *could* have, but unfortunately it is often used in conjunction with other fructose-containing sweeteners—commendable for lowering the overall fructose load, yet still off the table for us.[28]

I checked out the ten inches of shelf devoted to alternative sweeteners at our friendly neighborhood health food store and came up with two promising possibilities: agave and brown rice syrup.

---

[28]It's kind of amazing how many things we *didn't* learn till after our Year of No Sugar was over. It was then that our local health food store began carrying actual jars of barley malt syrup (wait! we can *buy* it?!), which fast became a favorite ingredient of mine when a recipe called for a thick, viscous sweetener such as honey or molasses.

Agave was the first in line. A sweetener derived from a Mexican perennial succulent, similar to ornamental Yucca plants, I had friends who swore by it. Plus, agave had been getting a lot of press lately as being the "healthy sweetener." I was curious but circumspect: could this really be the new wonder sweetener? The fact that agave was usually found marketed in the form of "syrup" or "nectar" sounded like a red flag, but for us, all it really came down to was one question: did it contain fructose? Or not?

The short answer is that agave *does* contain fructose—and how. Whereas you might recall that table sugar and high-fructose corn syrup contain in the neighborhood of 50 percent fructose and 50 percent glucose, agave syrup can contain as much as *90 percent fructose*. Remember how I said natural sweeteners *could be worse* for you than table sugar? Ladies and gentlemen, I give you: agave! Amazingly, agave is often recommended to diabetics as being glycemically neutral, meaning it does not raise one's blood sugar. Pop quiz! And *why* doesn't it raise blood sugar, class?

Because fructose, as we now know, is the stealth food. You'll recall the problem: fructose doesn't trigger the release of insulin (great!) because it's too busy traveling directly to the liver (bad!). There, for lack of anything better to do with it, the liver gets rid of it by creating lots of fatty acids that will then swim around in your bloodstream and block the insulin from delivering the glucose (the good stuff! energy of life!) to your cells. You'll recall my brilliant analogy of the traffic jam at rush hour and our friend Fred McInsulin. The whole reason diabetics have high insulin, folks, is because the fatty acids (read: fructose) are preventing the insulin from going where it needs to go. Eating MORE fructose may not raise your insulin levels right away, but it will create the fatty acids that will ultimately make it harder for the insulin to get where it needs to go, resulting in? That's right: higher insulin levels.[29]

So, to sum up, eating agave syrup instead of sugar seemed to me to be the equivalent of burning your house down before the tornado comes.[30] Agave syrup may be "natural" and "raw," but, you know, so is arsenic.[31]

Next on the shelf was brown rice syrup. Hmmmm, could we have *that*? "A sweetener derived by culturing cooked rice with enzymes," according to Wikipedia (which is surely never wrong), it's made up of "maltose, glucose, and maltotriose." Woo-hoo! There was no fructose in sight!

My friend Katrina weighed in: "Yeah, too bad it tastes like dog poo." *Oh*. Well. But then again she also thought our beloved Go Raw granola bars tasted like birdseed (like that's a *bad* thing!). I bought a jar of the sticky, amber-colored sweetener, and over the next few months, baked with it quite a bit. I found it became an invaluable tool in my baking arsenal, a very suitable substitute for similarly textured sweeteners, such as honey, molasses, and maple syrup. Although I wouldn't think of eating the stuff by the *spoonful*, it definitely didn't taste like dog poo. Not that I would know.

---

[29]In his book *Sweet Poison*, David Gillespie describes the abrupt about-face the American Diabetic Association did in 2002 when they realized recommending that diabetics sweeten with pure fructose was not only not good, but was in fact, dangerous, for this very reason. Gillespie, *Sweet Poison*, 60.

[30]The only good reason I've heard yet for favoring agave is that it can be easier to digest than some other sweeteners, for those who have digestion issues.

[31]Still, I wondered—was there a form of agave which included the plant fiber, meaning one could have the sweetness along with the original fiber, like eating an apple? Turns out no, unless you consider razor strops or hand soap (two of the uses for the non-sap parts of the plant) edible. Too bad.

So we were all getting along pretty well, drinking our sparkling water, eating our raisin granola bars, and baking with brown rice syrup when it came about that for several days I wasn't feeling so well, and as a result, I was getting behind—behind on my cooking, behind on my shopping, behind on my meal planning. Somehow we were muddling through, but one night, when I was feeling particularly desperate, half-ill and starving, I hauled out from the back of our freezer an industrial-size bag of frozen Bertolli chicken with cream sauce and bow tie pasta. Yes, the ingredient list was longer than my arm and appeared to have been at least partially written in some unknown foreign language, but this was a food emergency. At least there was no sugar, I reasoned, since I had purchased this on my first no-sugar run to BJ's a few weeks before.

But of course, silly me had to *double check*, which, if you are on No Sugar, can be a big mistake if you'd like to actually eat anytime in the near future. What I found in the fine print, in microscopic parenthesis, under a sub-ingredient listing for chicken "seasoning," was *that word* again: *dextrose*. Dextrose?
%^&*#$!

Remember the Panera salad dextrose? I had since encountered dextrose in other places, such as in the all-important French fries they sell at the ice-skating rink, but I had nonetheless been remiss in figuring this one out. I still didn't know *what the heck it was*...sugar? Not sugar? Fructose containing? No fructose? Was there no end to these intimidating, scientific "food" words? Grrrrrrrr....

But right then, at that *particular* moment, I felt crappy. I was hungry enough to eat a goat. And there was pretty much nothing else in the kitchen at that moment that seemed even remotely appealing. So I cut open the bag, dumped it into the pan, cooked it for the requisite ten minutes, and we ate it... mysterious dextrose or no.

Upon completing our meal, my first thought was that something was...*amiss*. What was it? It seemed really odd to me how quickly our meal had come together—I mean, a meal like chicken and bow tie pasta with spinach and cream sauce doesn't just happen all by itself! How long would a recipe like that normally take me? At least an hour but very likely more. Not to mention all the dirty dishes that would result from washing spinach, separately cooking chicken, carefully simmering the cream sauce in a pan while boiling the pasta in another pot...

It occurred to me that this meal had been sponsored: Brought To You By Dextrose! (As well as its friends Isolated Soy Protein Product and Sodium Phosphate!) The inverse correlation was very clear: the fewer chemicals and additives, the greater amount of meal prep/cooking and cleanup time, and vice versa.

But it had also become clear to me that I seriously needed to do some homework. When I looked up "dextrose" on the Internet, I found a host of confusing answers: "Better known today as glucose, this sugar is the chief source of energy in the body." Okaaaaay. Some sites defined dextrose as "corn sugar" that is "30 percent less sweet than pure or refined sugar." Okaaaaay. I was feeling pretty dense. Which was it? Is dextrose something that is generated in our bodies to provide energy, *or* is it an added sugar?

True confessions time: biochemistry was not my best subject. Sure, I knew some things about the suffix -*ose*. Thanks to "Sugar: The Bitter Truth," I knew the differences between terms like *su*crose, *glu*cose, and *fru*ctose: that glucose was the energy your cells use to function throughout your body; that sucrose was table sugar, a combination of equal parts glucose and fructose; that fructose, of course, was the root of all evil in the known universe and the spawn of the Evil Emperor from planet Naboo. But where the heck did *dextrose* come in?

Lucky for me I had someone who I could ask, someone who I considered to be the ultimate authority on all things fructose: Dr. Robert Lustig himself, the man behind "Sugar: The Bitter Truth," the very man who had inspired all our gastronomic shenanigans in the first place.

Bear in mind, however, that I have never met Dr. Lustig—I was, and continue to be, one more nutcase who happened to dig up his email address online in order to ask him all kinds of strange and annoying questions. The amazing thing is—he answered them. The first time I communicated with Dr. Lustig was before we began the No-Sugar Year. I wrote to tell him about our upcoming project and to ask him some questions, which I now see as incredibly stupid in retrospect—did wine contain fructose? What about honey? Duh! The patient man, he answered. And after that, I left him alone. For one thing, I was totally intimidated. I mean, he had *over a million* YouTube hits![32] He must've had about twelve thousand things more important to do than answer my idiotic questions—he probably had to go consult with NASA or appear on *Dancing with the Stars* or something! He probably had to go meet with

---

[32] At that time. After our Year of No Sugar was over, "Sugar: The Bitter Truth" would surpass two million hits on YouTube—and the last time I checked it was beyond 3.5 million. Not bad for a medical lecture!

the First Lady to talk about reducing the amount of fructose in the White House complimentary *mints* or something!

But I could see that this dextrose question wasn't going away, and I just wasn't confident I was going to get this one right by myself. After all, my one and only ten-minute, convenience-food dinner was riding on this. Lustig wrote me back—no doubt from the Situation Room—and kindly responded that dextrose is made from corn and that, essentially, "dextrose *is* glucose," and therefore for our fructose-free purposes, fine.

!!

It was *really* nice. In fact, I'd even go so far as to say really, really, *really* nice to have at least one "what about?" question end with a *definitive* "why, yes, you *can* have that!" even if it *was* dextrose and not, you know, hot fudge sundaes.

Later I would come to realize that this dextrose question was far, far more important than whether we could eat farfalle with spinach and cream sauce when the cook was feeling listless. Soon after getting Dr. Lustig's response, I read a book that was to change my life—and our year—again, called *Sweet Poison*, written by an Australian author named David Gillespie.

In it, Gillespie told a story I had now become familiar with: the story of fructose. If you've read the foreword to this book, you already know his story: once upon a time, there was a lawyer who was the father of four children, when one day his wife announced she was having twins. Gillespie, at that time, was overweight, unenergetic, and now, with the knowledge that he was soon to be father to a solid *half-dozen* progeny, completely petrified. *How on earth am I going to keep up with my kids?* he thought. Although he had tried every diet he could think of, he had never succeeded in finding a plan that worked, long term, for maintaining a healthy weight. Why is it, he wondered, that exercise and diets don't seem to *work*? Why is it that our ancestors never had this problem? What's the key difference between the way people once ate and the way we eat now that makes all the difference?

He was determined to figure it out, and figure it out he did. After piecing together mountains of research, Gillespie ultimately made the decision to try one thing, just one: eliminate added fructose from his diet. In doing so he lost ninety pounds. Today, not only do he and his family abstain from sugar, but so do countless other friends, acquaintances, and members of his community around him, who were convinced simply by observing Gillespie's dramatic transformation.[33]

If watching "The Bitter Truth" had turned on the a-ha lightbulb in my brain, reading *Sweet Poison* turned on a second lightbulb, one that filled in the details where before there had been shadow. A non-doctor, Gillespie has a terrific knack for translating all the various medical findings and research into accurate but comprehensible layperson speak. He is also, incidentally, very funny, which can be helpful when you're hanging in there by your fingernails talking about phosphofructokinase 1 and the islets of Langerhans.

I enjoyed the book immensely and felt a great sense of confirmation in what we were doing. Maybe—just maybe—we

---

[33]Since the publication of Gillespie's *Sweet Poison*, he has gone on to become a tireless advocate of No Sugar in Australia, appearing regularly on television, radio, and in print, in addition to writing another book on the subject *The Sweet Poison Quit Plan* and maintaining an informative website and blog. It would not be an exaggeration to say he is the father of a burgeoning No-Sugar movement in Australia.

weren't entirely insane. But just as significant for me would be the discovery Gillespie had made with regard to cooking because what he had happened upon was the idea of using *powdered dextrose in cooking*. Powdered dextrose? I had never heard of such a thing. Heck, it wasn't even on the alternative sweeteners micro-shelf at Nature's Market! This was truly uncharted territory and I began to wonder: how weird was this really gonna be?

Following Gillespie's instructions in the book, I ordered a twenty-pound container of the fine white powder. *Could this be?* I wondered. *Could we really have a dessert that didn't have sugar in it* or *taste like bananas? And was actually* good? I fairly salivated at the prospect. At last the box arrived and it was…enormous! The orange plastic jar was roughly the size of a beach ball and was packaged similar to those colossal jars of weight-gain powder you see in vitamin stores. Seriously? I wondered…

Spurred on by what was left of my poor, neglected sweet tooth, I tackled David's recipe for Strawberry Ricotta Cheesecake. I was fully prepared to be deeply disappointed. I reminded the kids this was an experiment and might not be as wonderfully delicious as the name might suggest. But it did *look* pretty great in the oven, rising and browning just a bit on the top…and the smell was a warm, faint strawberry-inflected sweetness, *distinctly* dessert-y.

It cooled on the stove and sank a bit while we had dinner. After dinner, I eyed the cheesecake with great trepidation before finally cutting into it and distributing the plates. It sure did *look* good but…

One bite, however, and my skepticism evaporated. In its place appeared surprise—also, delight. I smiled big. I looked around and saw that the kids were smiling big too—in between big bites of white fluffy dessert, dessert that contained *no fructose...no added sugar*. And it was GOOD! *Really* good!

If this was a made-for-TV movie, this would have been the exact moment that the soundtrack featuring the hallelujah chorus would break in, playing jubilantly over jump cuts of us stuffing our faces. I couldn't stop exclaiming how *good* it really was! I mean, it wasn't *S-W-E-E-T* but it was quietly *sweet*—which, it seemed, we were starting to prefer anyway. We all polished off our plates. The kids immediately were getting ideas: could we make ice cream with dextrose? How about sugar cookies?

A new world had opened.

We had found something to bake with, without the toxic effects to our bodies of fructose and without endangering the world's supply of bananas. What more could we possibly ask for? Well, I'll give you one word: chocolate.

Sure, we had our Ovaltine, which was a decent hot chocolate stand-in, and I could even make a delicious brownie now that we had dextrose to mix with the cocoa, but *actual* chocolate was one thing we just were not going to get. Or so we thought.

And then one day Steve came home with a shiny, foil-wrapped bar. It looked an awful lot like my long-lost friend chocolate, and I felt sinful just looking at the thing. I gasped and averted my eyes.

But, "No!" he said. "Look—*we can eat this*."

Now, when your name is Eve, you tend to be a little wary

of temptation scenarios, so I eyed my husband keenly. In my desperation to find sweet substitutes that our Year of No Sugar could accommodate, I thought I had seen it all. Could it possibly be there was something I had missed?

ChocoPerfection was the name, with the tag line "Sugar Free…Naturally!" If it was good—which I highly doubted— how could it possibly be okay? Upon hearing of our project, our friend Ellen had given the bar to Steve.

"I," she had said ominously, "am about to change your life."

We eyed the gold wrapper. We read the ingredients. We reread the ingredients. There were two I wasn't familiar with: oligofructose and erythritol. Hmmmm. Sounded suspicious. I looked it up. Turns out, oligofructose is extracted from fruits or vegetables—in this case from chicory root. It is touted as being not only *not bad*, but it is, in fact, health promoting on account of the extremely high amount of dietary fiber (one ChocoPerfection bar brings with it an astounding 52 percent of recommended dietary fiber) as well as "probiotic" effects— which is to say it is believed to stimulate the growth of good bacteria in the colon.

Then we have erythritol. I found out that it is a "sugar alcohol," which generally isn't such a good thing, since sugar alcohols such as xylitol and Maltitol are known to be associated with laxative properties and "gastric distress." Ew! However, according to unerring wisdom of the Internet, erythritol is unique: unlike other sugar alcohols, it is absorbed in the small intestine and then excreted. Translation? *No* tummy troubles.

The upshot was that, together, oligofructose and erythritol might just have a pretty good thing going. They supplement one another's sweetness and counteract one another's aftertaste. There were only two downsides that I could see, and they didn't appear to be deal breakers: firstly, after we tried our bar from Ellen, I found that that boatload of fiber made my tummy gurgly. Now, could I live with that if it meant I could have real (tasting) chocolate? Yes, sir, yes, sir, three bags full. My second complaint was its expense: one tiny 1.8-ounce bar goes for between three and four dollars— nearly a dollar a bite. Again, if that meant I could have an actual (tasting) authentic (seeming) bona fide (your results may vary) *chocolate bar* once in a while during our long, long, LONG Year of No Sugar? Pardon me while I go mortgage the house. I have chocolate to buy, people.

Just like with dextrose powder, we would have to order these bars online. (We had entered the Land of Extreme Groceries, apparently.) That's when we found out that the same company also made a granular "sugar" for use in baking. At forty some dollars a pound, it wasn't exactly going to make the folks at Domino quake in their sugar-encrusted boots, but to us it sounded like we might just have hit the jackpot. We placed an order for a batch of the dollar-per-bite bars and one *very* pricey little bag of "sugar."

When our package at last arrived, it didn't take long to realize that the faux sugar was a bit of a disappointment. We tried a few test batches of peanut butter cookies and found that the texture was off—a little too crunchy, dry, and grainy—plus there was a distinct aftertaste to it. The bars, however, were just like that first one we had tried: good. Not amazing but *good*. In fact, they were just chocolate-like enough that we actually felt like we were cheating.

Which was actually a good point: *were* we cheating? The more I thought about it, the more I just felt…*weird* about the whole idea. I couldn't help but feel that somehow this was not entirely okay.

I tried to puzzle it out: from everything I could discern, oligofructose and erythritol *don't* turn to fat in your bloodstream, *don't* raise blood sugar levels, and *don't* even cause hammer toes. I wondered: Is this an artificial sweetener because it isn't sucrose/fructose, or is it a natural sweetener because it comes from chicory root? If the point is to avoid fructose, as well as artificial sweeteners that have known negative effects on the body, then we *were* doing that! If the point is to avoid not only extracted fructose, but any stuff that *simulates* fructose, then we *weren't* doing that! Help!

I felt so conflicted and confused that once again I emailed my question to Dr. Lustig and waited breathlessly for—at last!—a definitive answer. What he graciously sent me, instead, was this:

"As to non-nutritive sweeteners, there are pharmacokinetics (what your body does to a drug) and pharmacodynamics (what a drug does to your body). We have the former (that's how they got FDA approval), but none of the latter. So I can't recommend any of them. But stay tuned, this information may be coming in the future."

Hmm. Well, that's essentially where I had ended up before: I don't know. The thing I realized is that Dr. Lustig is a doctor and I'm a writer; he was offering a doctor answer to what was, for me, a writer question.

So I kept searching. I returned to my other big inspiration: David Gillespie had this to say in his book *Sweet Poison*:

No amount of rat studies will reassure me that industrial chemicals that have been in our food supply for less than a few decades are definitely safe…It took almost one hundred years of mass consumption before researchers started questioning whether sugar was dangerous. Can we really know if sucralose or aspartame are safe after just a few decades?

Hmm again. I was getting closer to an answer. Gillespie wasn't talking about oligofructose, per se, but as Lustig had pointed out, *all* these new sweetening options are big question marks at this point. And question marks, Gillespie reminds us, don't have a terrific track record when it comes to our bodies' health.

But back to ethics: it still just felt like cheating to me. Steve was a big ChocoPerfection fan and much less conflicted about the whole thing than I was. His argument was that even with our special chocolate bars, spending a year avoiding all added sugar was still really, *really* hard. Which is true. And yet, don't you just have to go with your gut, so to speak?

So we slowly, *slowly* finished off the special chocolate bars and decided not to order more. The bag of "sugar" was shoved to the back of the pantry shelf. Sigh.

Banana, anyone?

CHAPTER 8

POOP DOESN'T LIE

I don't mean to be indelicate, folks, but I think the time has come to talk about one of the *other* consequences of eating. As one of our children's books puts it: "just about every animal poops."

Quite honestly, I never used to give poop a lot of thought. As a teenager, I attended a summer horse camp where we spent large portions of our day managing the unmentionable stuff, shoveling and carting it around, climbing small mountains of it in order to get to the designated wheelbarrow-dump-out spot, trying to get away with ditching it instead in the bushes or behind a stack of old moldy hay. But it wasn't until I first went to a local chiropractor for pregnant-lady back pain about ten years ago that I was given a reason to think about the issue of poop as a matter of *health*, rather than mere inconvenience, necessity, or proper horse care.

"About how often do you have a bowel movement?" Ray asked me. Ray Foster is not only a wonderful chiropractor, but also a neighbor and fellow parent. I was more than a little mortified to be asked such an unmentionable question, not to mention the fact that I really had no idea how to answer it. I had to admit—I really didn't *know*. Certainly not every day, *maybe* every couple of days…heck, who knows? For all I knew, it could've been once every *month*. Are we really supposed to keep track of such things? I wondered. Had I missed that day in health class? Sure, I remember learning the four food groups (I had always enjoyed the fact that there was a fifth, "other" category for all the really interesting things like Pop Rocks and Crisco), but did we ever, *ever* talk about what happened to those foods after they entered the big melting pot of our digestive system? About the *other* side of eating?

Definitely not. I imagine the prospect of having to tackle yet another giggle-fest topic in high school health class was just too much for our beleaguered teachers. I wonder if I had had a greater sense of nutritional intelligence, would it have swayed me from following a path of uninformed vegetarianism for two decades? Now, I know this is a *gargantuan* tangent, but hang in there—I promise this all comes back around to poop.

Beginning at age fourteen, back when this was still a fairly unheard-of practice among my peers, I officially became Some Kind of Vegetarian. Part of a protracted and somewhat naïve attempt to express my love for animals, I evolved slowly over the years through a rainbow of vegetarian-y shades: no red meat, no poultry, no fish…I never made it all the way to vegan. (The idea of giving up my beloved cheese plainly horrified me—"What, no *nachos*?")

The fact that my parents both thought it a passing teenage fancy surely made my commitment all the more steadfast. I was asserting my independence in the arena of food (this sounds familiar, somehow…), but there was one little problem. I was eating like *crap*.

Of course, as a young adult this didn't bother me a bit—I loved animals and abhorred the thought of their mass slaughter in food factories. At the time terms like *free range* and *organic* had yet to make their way into the national consciousness, so eating animals—as far as any of us knew—by definition involved animal cruelty. I was way more interested in not being a nutritional hypocrite than in eating healthily—whatever *that* meant. After all, society kept changing its mind radically on what constituted "healthy eating" anyway...right? I just figured I would eat what was appealing and my body would sort everything out. I reveled in the idea that I was eating according to a higher moral ideal: what you don't kill makes you stronger. I mean, I was saving *animals*, for crying out loud!

The problem was, I was what they call a "French fry vegetarian." Don't ever let anyone tell you that vegetarians are by definition healthier than meat eaters—this is a common misconception. Just because someone doesn't eat meat doesn't mean they subsist on sustainably harvested seaweed chips and free-trade kale. Let's just say, we might also label this extended period of my life the "Pizza and Grilled Cheese Era." (You can see why I would've made a miserable vegan.)

During those years, I simply ate *around* the meat everywhere I went and enjoyed more than my share of all the non-meat items on the menu: cheese, bread, pasta, more cheese. To my mother's dismay, I thought nothing of regularly having a bagel with cream cheese for dinner. Once in a blue moon, I might eat a vegetable, just for the sheer novelty of it.

At that rate, it's a wonder I didn't just stop "emitting" altogether. (See? Poop!) I probably would've made it to my fiftieth birthday party and then, at the height of the festivities, exploded. But somehow the human body makes do—or poo—with what it's given. Lucky for me, my husband convinced me eating meat might help my low-energy problem, from which I had suffered for years—and you know what? He was right. Gradually, over time, I found out that the more meat I ate, the better I felt. At long last, after twenty years, my "higher moral ideals" gave way to a rather novel idea: *feeling healthier.*

Which isn't to say that I was *healthy*. But I was health*ier*, which was a good place to start. I was happier, more energetic, and way less prone to sudden, debilitating attacks of I-feel-crappy.

After twenty years of vegi-something-ism and my subsequent foray back into the carnivorous universe, I felt pretty good. I still wished I had more energy, could find time for more sleep and regular exercise, and all those good things we all say we want but rarely get around to doing anything about. I cooked a lot, more than most folks I knew, so I figured that was as much as I could do in the health department. And then came Dr. Lustig and his darned extremely convincing argument. So the obvious question was going to be, after embarking on an adventure aimed at being healthier, *were* we healthier?

Everyone kept wanting to know. Every time we talked about the No-Sugar Project, even after only a few weeks, people wanted to know: Have you lost weight? Do you feel better? Do the kids seem happier/healthier/calmer? I wondered, *How* do *you quantify such an ambiguous thing as health?* About three months in to our year, I had not lost any weight, the kids didn't seem noticeably calmer, nor had my hair turned green or any other very obvious side effect. I did *think* I felt healthier, and I did *seem* to not get sick as often or for as long as I might otherwise—surely, there were all subjective issues which could just as easily be due to coincidence or a placebo effect. If we were going to notice any significant changes, it wasn't going to be in the first few days or weeks—I even wondered if we'd notice in a matter of months.

That's the thing about sugar: you're talking a long, long timeline. Sugar isn't crack; it doesn't cause you to get in a car accident or have a seizure or jump off a rooftop or anything dramatic or interesting like that. As we've seen, sugar's deleterious effects are insidious and long term. Remember how many decades we all struggled as a society just to admit what everyone pretty much already knew about *cigarettes*, i.e., that they were *bad* for you? Well, an analogy between cigarettes and sugar is an apt one: the majority of the damage in each is accomplished not with one use, or a few uses, but with continued steady use over years, decades. That's one reason why proving their connection with disease is so difficult.

Consequently, "better health" for us was simply not going to be a readily observable condition—much less provable—after one lousy year of not eating sugar. We couldn't claim to have cured ourselves of diabetes or prevented an impending heart attack or nipped a case of obesity in the bud. A year may seem like an eternity to us, but in the grand scheme of an average American lifetime? One year doesn't amount to a hill of beans. It was too bad, but most of our "evidence" was going to be highly subjective and largely anecdotal.

However, one thing that is simply *not* subjective is poop (see? I told you to hang in there), and I was more than a little embarrassed to notice that—apparently—I was full of it. At first, I had tried to ignore the obvious change, but the facts were as inescapable as they were mystifying to me: on our No Sugar Plan, I didn't just "emit" like clockwork; I pooped like a Swiss freaking watch. At *least* once a day. If not more. Compared to my vegetarian-ish days of God-knows-when-I-last-went, this new state of affairs was, well, hard to ignore.

What was going on *here?* I wondered. *Was* it the lack of sugar per se? Or could it be the fact that we were eating many more fruits to supplement sweetness in our diet? Could it simply be the fact that we were making so many more things from scratch in order to avoid sugar, and in doing so were also avoiding a host of other food additives and preservatives?

I really didn't know. All I knew was, suddenly my body was, well, *working* better than it had perhaps ever before, which was really, uh, nice. And probably a good sign of improved health. Not to be gross about it or anything.

Although the poop issue was evident almost immediately, as the year progressed, another, more subtle change became gradually but increasingly clear: our palates were changing.

As it turned out, our monthly sugar-containing dessert was good for another purpose besides staving off a family mutiny—it also served as a sort of de facto check-in point for our tongues. I suppose it speaks to my longtime love affair with sugar that it simply never *occurred* to me that, after abstaining from dessert for long stretches, when we finally got to have it, *we might not enjoy it.*

You heard me. Or, at least, we might not enjoy it as much as we once did or as much as we expected to. But believe it or not, there were moments when eating our oh-so-rare sugar treat became downright *unpleasant.* There came a point when I stopped looking forward to our monthly dessert and started dreading that too-sweet disruption of our now-familiar routine.

For example, while we delighted in those first few, eagerly anticipated treats in January and February, by April, I began to notice that our monthly treat now gave me a headache and a racing pulse, not to mention a weird, syrupy taste in my mouth that made me want to go brush my teeth. Huh. In August we encountered the first monthly dessert that none of us would finish, and by September the elaborate concoction I created for Steve's birthday actually made me feel quite ill.

As I lay on the couch with a pounding headache and feeling awful, it occurred to me that perhaps I should be worried. I had wanted to do an experiment, sure, be healthier, yes, but had I intended to give my family a sweet-ectomy? Never.

I had read about this, in David Gillespie's book. He said it took time, but within a few weeks of avoiding sugar, one begins to lose the taste for it—it simply ceases to be appealing. He was right, of course, but what I was discovering was that for me it was a teeny bit more complicated than that. Whereas my *tongue* didn't want that piece of banana cream pie or cone of gelato, my *brain* still did.

What ensued was a sort of worst-case scenario in which I looked forward to our dessert night for weeks on end until finally, at long last, I'd have the opportunity to enjoy it and... it tasted *awful*. It reminded me of that phenomenon when I was pregnant and all chocolate turned to sawdust in my mouth—it was frustrating. Disappointing. Maddening. But it was fascinating too. Clearly we were on the right track—things were *happening* in our bodies, our senses were *changing*. It's just that if that particular track meant I'd never again enjoy a nice piece of rhubarb pie—*ever*—well, I just wasn't sure my brain would ever forgive me.

The only other indicator I found which was somewhat measurable would come at the end of our year. It was then that it occurred to me to compare our kids' report cards, listing their absences for the trimester. After subtracting the days I knew had been missed for non-illness reasons, such as travel,[34] what I came up with I found kind of fascinating. Look:

SCHOOL ABSENCES BY TRIMESTER					
	Trimester One (Fall)		Trimester Two (Winter)	Trimester Three (Spring)	Year Total
	Quarter One	Quarter Two	Quarter Three	Quarter Four	
Greta Absences					
pre-K[35]	–	–	–	–	??
kindergarten	2	5	5	5	17
first grade[36]	3	4	1	3	11
second grade	0	5		1	6
third grade	9	2		0	11
fourth grade	0	3		7	10
fifth grade	5	1		0	6
sixth grade	1	0		2	3
Ilsa Absences					
pre-K	–		–	–	15
kindergarten	5		1	2	8
first grade	0		6	4	10

[34]For example, in third grade, I know Greta missed the one and only week when they were taught fractions because we chose that week to bring the girls to Tuscany where we learned how to make fresh pasta and cook rabbit from a friend's honest-to-goodness Italian mama. Consequently, Greta has never missed an opportunity to remind me of this fact whenever fractions appear on her math homework. (Would it be wrong of me to suggest that knowing how to make gnocchi might be almost as important?)

I've indicated the trimesters during which we were doing the No Sugar Project in bold. As you can see, during our No-Sugar Year, Greta missed only two school days and Ilsa only three. *Well*, that's *pretty good*, I thought. Then I decided to look at the last third of our No-Sugar Year—during which we could be presumed to be enjoying the maximum cumulative health benefits of our year. I compared their fall absences from the previous year (2010) to those of fall 2011, our Year of No Sugar—(see bolded numbers). I noticed that from one fall to the next, they had each gone from five absences to either one (Greta) or zero (Ilsa).

Zero? Zero.

I decided to look further back—I mean this *is* elementary school, folks. Club Med for germs! Every year we, like all the other families we know, run the gauntlet of flus, head colds, wracking coughs, and of course the dreaded stomach viruses. Usually we're happy if we've managed to avoid some reasonable portion of the illness smorgasbord. I wondered, had we *ever* had a trimester with *no* absences? Turns out we had, more than once, so that big, fat zero fact wasn't as impressive in and of itself as I might've hoped.

But I found a few more interesting statistics. The school year, of course, doesn't coincide with the calendar year, or, consequently, our Year of No Sugar. What if we compared school absences during calendar years?

Hmmmmm. Because I like charts, I made another one:

---

[35]For pre-K absences, I had no record, since there are no report cards at that level. Through the detective work of some very accommodating school officials I was able to obtain Ilsa's records, albeit without breakdown within the year.

[36]During Greta's kindergarten through first grade the school was on a different, quarterly system.

SCHOOL ABSENCES BY CALENDAR YEAR		
	Ilsa	Greta
2007	n/a	8 approx.[37]
2008	n/a	15
2009	n/a	2
2010	between 5 and 20	15
2011	3	2

As we've noted, during all of 2011—the all-important Year of No Sugar—Greta missed only two days of school and Ilsa three; so what about other years? In 2009, Greta had the same number of sick days (2) as during our No-Sugar Year—not so remarkable. However, in both 2008 and 2010 Greta missed fifteen days of school—an increase over our Year of No Sugar of um…650 percent.

Because Ilsa is younger, of course, we have less data to work with, and because we don't have Ilsa's pre-K absences broken down into trimesters, we can't say exactly how many absences occurred in 2010 versus 2009. We do know that the number of absences she had in 2010 would be at least five and at most twenty. This indicates an increase over our Year of No Sugar of falling somewhere between 67 and 567 percent. If we decide to compromise and meet in the middle (which we can do since I'm clearly a terrible scientist), we might say Ilsa very likely had somewhere in the neighborhood of 250 percent increase of absences in the year prior to No Sugar.

Now, did we have the occasional sore throat or sniffle during our year? Sure. So I can't say that eating no added sugar

---

[37] The quarterly system makes it difficult to tell precisely.

made us into Super Family who could leap over nasty viruses with a single bound.

But I *can* say that if you look at the numbers, it suuuuuure does look like our kids were comparatively quite healthy during our No-Sugar Year—*and* that they were noticeably health*ier* during 2011 than two out of the previous three years.

So there you have it. The physical evidence of our No-Sugar Year came down to three *P*s: Poop, Palate, and Presence (as opposed to absence? From school? Aw, c'mon!). Anecdotal? Circumstantial? Perhaps. But nothing to sneeze at.

I did promise them I wouldn't make a chart about their poops, though.

CHAPTER 9

BUT WHAT ABOUT
THE *KIDS*?

Now, with all this talk about sugar equaling love, or getting confused with love, it's kind of inevitable that a lot of folks would see denying a kid their God-given, American-sized portion of sugar as stopping just short of child abuse.

Inevitably, the aspect of our project that people found most compelling was the fact that the children were *doing it too*. And the questions they asked most often had to do with the children:

"How are they *taking* it?"

"Are they freaking out?"

"Do they act calmer without sugar?"

"How do you *do* it?"

The answers were often complex: Some days the kids adored the project, acting as if it was something significant and wonderful—something that bound us together and made our family unique; other times they'd rail against me and the project for totally ruining their lives, or make maudlin faces at the prospect of being in the vicinity of a treat they knew full well they were not going to be able to have.

But when I say "kids," I really mean Greta, because Ilsa,

at age six, was really the more easygoing of the two when it came to, well, everything.

Greta, on the other hand, as an ideal teenager-in-training, tends toward the dramatic and is doing an excellent job living up to the legacy of her name (as in Garbo). Early on she made a point everywhere we went to announce to anyone within hearing range the specifics of our project, to which the usual response would be a puzzled, piteous grown-up look that seemed to say, "You poor thing, you have controlling hippie parents don't you? Do they make you eat lima beans for breakfast?"

Even though I was pretty sure my kids would survive the year relatively untraumatized, like most parents, I still agonized. Would they ever forgive me? Would they grow up feeling deprived and alienated? Would they one day hoard sweets in their shoe closet?

But I forged on. I learned quickly NOT to take them with me to the supermarket so they could drool over all the lovely products in shiny packages that we weren't buying. I became big on after-school snacks like popcorn and hummus and my latest attempt at a decent no-sugar cookie. I learned to pay $1.50 for an apple at the ice-skating rink snack bar, even though the apples and other snacks we brought from home were exponentially better *and* cheaper.

"It's more *fun* to buy it here, Mommy," Ilsa illuminated me. *Okay*, I thought. We weren't buying the soft pretzels or hot cocoa or French fries or Gatorade that everyone else was, but at least we could buy something from the concession stand too—and I realized that when my kids were feeling deprived, that $1.50 apple could make all the difference.

Now, let me just say this right up front: I love our elementary school. I adore it. I want to marry it. Starting when Greta was in pre-K, we'd been attending this school for six years now and have enjoyed every minute of the warm, welcoming community of learning it provides—no kidding. I wish *I* had gone to a school this good as a kid. In the past, they have even done great things on the healthy food front, such as plant a school garden and invite parents to contribute their favorite soup recipes for lunch. Currently there's even a grant-funded healthy snack program that gives the kids fruits and vegetables in between meals.

————————

Mom says that at home we can't eat sugar, period. But at school and at other places it's our choice. Like today at school, we had an all school read and everyone in the school was offered hot chocolate. My teacher gave us each a marshmallow and it was my friend's birthday and she brought in chocolate-covered marshmallows. Of course, I thought about it carefully and decided to take it. But whoa, my friend Sara made beignets (ben-yahs) and shared them with our class. Not wanting to be left out I grabbed one from the tray before it was passed to the next table. I knew I had not broken any rules because mom said it was my choice outside of the home. Many times I've felt guilt. And many times my mom has had to assure me "it's your choice and you've done nothing wrong." But today I think I achieved a goal because after I had the sweets I didn't feel bad. I think I know why. Because I was in a situation that I was able to make the right decision for me at that time. So my point here is we all make our own choices. And just because I'm not following one rule at one specific moment, that doesn't mean I won't be in a minute. And also that I'm not following another rule.

—from Greta's journal

———————

Unfortunately, none of this alters the fact that the school food, the day-to-day menu, is *packed* with added sugar. Even I, who had been focusing on the added-sugar issue with a myopic vengeance since the turn of the year, was shocked one day when, out of curiosity, I sat down to really *look* at the breakfast menu that regularly came home in backpacks with a slew of other color-coded papers.

Once again, though, there was a certain amount of decoding involved. When they say "assorted whole-grain cereal" read: Frosted Flakes. When they say "Nutri-Grain fruit bar" read: high-fructose corn syrup. When they say "graham crackers" read: crystalline fructose (or lab fructose—the sweetest ingredient our food scientists have managed to come up with to date. Think: sugar heroin).

So, I decided to get out my highlighter. I counted a total of thirty possible options on the breakfast menu including condiments and syrup; out of those thirty items, eighteen had added sugar—*more than half.* But it got worse.

Looking closer, the school menu advertises "Milk Variety Is Served with Every Meal!" What does "milk variety" mean? This means *chocolate* milk. Okay, so if we assume a child chooses *chocolate* milk with his or her breakfast every morning, we are now up to *twenty-four* items out of thirty possible breakfast choices, or *eighty percent of breakfast items containing added sugar.*

And then there's this: every day children having breakfast are given a piece of fresh fruit. Of course, the fruit has fructose in it too—although, as we know, eating it with the corresponding fiber and micronutrients, they're at least effectively balancing that portion of fructose out. So while it isn't added sugar, per se, it is still yet even *more sugar*.

Therefore, if we are looking at the number of items containing fructose (read: poison) in our breakfast menu for March 2011, and assuming a choice of chocolate milk every day? We can now bring our total of items containing sugar/fructose to *twenty-nine out of thirty, or roughly 97 percent*. What is the one item left *not* containing fructose? Cream cheese for our bagel on Tuesday.

This isn't atypical for breakfast in general, which, as we know, wins the award for "Meal Most Likely to Contain Tons of Sugar When You Least Expect It." In fact, one of David Gillespie's five cardinal rules for avoiding fructose is "Be Careful at Breakfast." Oooo! That sounds ominous, like a horror movie for diabetics.

All this being said, I know the arguments: "some breakfast is better than no breakfast at all," and "my kid won't drink milk if it isn't chocolate." Personally, I don't buy this. Part of the problem is that as parents and as a society, we are providing too many choices.[38] Did Laura Ingalls refuse to drink her milk if it wasn't chocolate? To eat her cereal if it didn't have Day-Glo marshmallows in it? I have to believe that, if your kid is hungry enough, they'll eat. If they're thirsty enough, they'll drink. Are Frosted Flakes and Lucky Charms *really* the best we can do? I know that the school valiantly puts up with all us

---

[38]Or as I've mentioned before, the *illusion* of choices.

demanding parents, each of whom wants or expects something different; I know if the school had to pay attention to *every* parent's pet peeve concern we'd probably have to cancel school altogether until we could figure out how to encase each child in a nice firm bubble. Still, I cringe when I read the wrappers that I dig from the bottom of my kids' backpacks and learn about the high-fructose corn syrup in their Rice Krispies, the partially-hydrogenated vegetable shortening in their Goldfish Grahams, and lovely sounding things like methylcellulose, diglycerides, and something called "propylene glycol esters of fatty acids" in their Nutri-Grain bars. Yum.

And, yes, those wrappers *were* still coming home, at least in one child's backpack. You see, although I provided the kids breakfasts at home and packed their lunches, Ilsa was fond of having breakfast *again* once she got to school. Sometimes this meant an apple and milk (fine), and other times this meant I found the dreaded *wrappers*.

So I redoubled my efforts. Whereas once upon a time I would've sleepily thrown three or four cereal boxes on the table with some bowls, now I was actively planning a loose breakfast rotation: soft boiled eggs and toast,[39] plain yogurt with strawberries, oatmeal with bananas, toast with cheese and cantaloupe, bagels[40] and cream cheese with slices of orange. Occasionally I'd brew some peppermint tea for the girls or have Steve make up the frothy milk drink called a steamer (which we grew to love back when we used to make it with maple syrup), or a warm mug of Ovaltine.

---

[39]From homemade, no-sugar bread.

[40]*Supermarket* bagels contain added sugar, but those of our local bagel shop, as it turned out, did not.

And in fact, Ilsa *was* trying. She actually told me she had been asking the breakfast ladies if the Rice Krispies had sugar in them and that they had told her "no" or "not really" or something along those lines. Ilsa knew a lot more about fructose than the average six-year-old, but the specifics of products with ingredient lists got murky fast, and in fact, who *aren't* they confusing for nowadays? She was doing what we all were—asking. And just like for us, some answers were more, well, *helpful* than others.

So, did I *forbid* Ilsa from getting snacks from the breakfast ladies in the morning? I did not. We talked periodically about the food choices she made while not at home. She got it. She tried to figure it out for her particular first-grade level of understanding of the project. She did her best—and then she let it go.

I couldn't have asked a single thing more of her.

––––––––

We were very nearly halfway through our year when Greta and I did a short presentation for her fifth-grade class we might've titled "Yeah, like, What the Heck Is Greta's Family Doing, Again?" I was nervous. I realized that for all the talking and reading and thinking and agonizing I'd done on this subject, I hadn't spoken before a group about it at all. Sure they were fifth graders, not a congressional inquiry, but nonetheless I had visions of sophisticated biochemistry questions being lobbed at me by kids who aren't about to give up their chocolate-covered Twinkies without a fight.

Worse, as I made up my notes for the talk, I struggled with striking the right chord somewhere in between being the world's most boring health teacher ("Can anyone tell me the incredibly fascinating difference between *lactose* and *galactose*? Hmmm?") and scaring the pee out of them ("Well, according to what I've been reading, sugar causes obesity, heart disease, liver disease, diabetes, prostate and breast cancer, not to mention elephantitis of the pores, rampant yellow toe fungus, the end of the world, *and* not getting asked to the junior prom!!! AIIGHHHH!")

Most of all, I worried about the same thing all mothers of preteen girls worry about: budding eating disorders. The last, last, LAST thing I wanted to do in the course of discussing important topics like the national epidemic of obesity was to inadvertently encourage some fifth-grade girl *not to eat*. Had I put enough pressure on myself yet?

But I think it went okay after all. I focused on some key terms and statistics I thought might perk their interest: How every man, woman, and child consumes on average 2.7 pounds of sugar per *week*. (I held up a five-pound bag of sugar to demonstrate one person's two-week allotment. Interestingly, the kids were utterly unfazed by this.) What a "Western Disease" is. (Guesses included pneumonia and malaria, so it was good we talked about this one.) And how doctors decide whether a person is a healthy weight, overweight, or obese. I mean, you hear about an "epidemic of obesity," but what does that really *mean*?

I put the BMI (Body Mass Index) formula on the board: weight in pounds times 703, divided by the square of your height in inches. Amazingly, the kids really perked up at this. There were sudden shuffling noises as kids grabbed for pieces of paper and pencils, presumably so they could calculate their own BMI, although I have to admit that I wasn't about to start figuring out what sixty-six squared is on paper.

I demonstrated how I got my own BMI by plugging in my own height and weight, and whipping out my calculator.

Yesterday the school served ice cream with pizza. And unfortunately I sit with three people that always have school lunch. Or almost always, 'cause one of them brought home lunch. But the other two were teasing him in a playful way saying, "You know you want it you know you do." And then eating it in front of our faces.

—from Greta's journal

The other most popular part of the hour was more predictable: when Greta distributed my most recent dextrose dessert effort: cocoa brownies. I was delighted to see that everyone ate their entire brownie—everyone!—which to me equals baking success. Heck, some of these kids may very well view sugar as its own food group. That's one of the things you can still say about kids at this age—they haven't learned to varnish their opinions yet in the name of politeness. Most fifth graders aren't about to eat a yucky brownie just to be polite to someone else's mom.

And then the talk was over. I'm not sure how much of it any of them actually retained, but I figured at least we started the conversation. If we managed to plant even one seed of an idea, then how great would that be?

If I had any fears that I was over-exaggerating the state of our current sugar-addiction epidemic, they were put to rest on the last day of school which, surprise! Abounded with sugar.

Exhibit A: Twizzler Math.

Not only do we love our daughters' school, but furthermore, we have been lucky enough to love every teacher either of our two daughters has had so far—which is really quite impressive. (By the time *I* got to sixth grade, I seem to recall having had my share of doozies in the teacher department, including Mr. Major who liked to have the girls sit on his lap and "give him some sugar." Oo! Do you think that's where this all started? Hmmmm.)

We especially loved Greta's fifth-grade teacher. Mrs. Roberts is the kind of teacher who seems to take each student under her wing in some protective, affectionate, almost aunt-like or grandmotherly way. To celebrate the end of the annual school-wide reading program, she invited the *entire fifth grade* over to her house for movies, a picnic, and swimming. I mean, can *I* retake fifth grade but have Mrs. Roberts this time?

Like any treasured aunt or beloved grandmother, Mrs. Roberts gives the kids treats—hot chocolate in the winter, candy at Halloween, Skittles if a kid is having a particularly hard day, and Twizzlers on the last day of school. But what astounded me on the last day of school wasn't the fact that Mrs. Roberts had given out Twizzlers, but rather the Hershey Company's savvy marketing of Twizzlers as a way to practice *fractions*. Yes, in fact, there was a whole book about it, which Mrs. Roberts was kind enough to let me flip through in my astonishment.

The book-directed exercise went something like this: if you have ten Twizzlers, and you eat three of them, what fraction represents the amount of Twizzlers you have left? Voilà! Twizzler math.

Really, the marketing possibilities are endless. Coming soon to a classroom near you: M&M's addition, Sour Patch subtraction, jelly bean geometry...

Exhibit B: The PTO picnic.

Actually, we did fairly well at the Last Day of School Picnic. Every year, each grade is assigned a food to bring, while the Parent Teacher Organization provides the volunteers and hot dogs. In addition to the dogs (probably okay, but being strict, hold the bun), there were chips (go for the Smartfood, skip the SunChips and Doritos), macaroni salads (skip these—mayo has sugar), tossed salads, watermelon, and chopped veggies (yay!). All in all, not a communal meal in which we need fear starving to death. Of course, there was dessert, and I had the watermelon while my kids opted for the little paper cups of ice cream,[41] but I did manage to steer them away from the lemonade and in the direction of water or milk, so I figured we had done *okay*.

But a funny thing happened. In addition to my green salad contribution, I brought along a bottle of my homemade lemon juice and olive oil salad dressing, mainly for our family's benefit. I placed the bottle on the table with a whole regiment of other bottles, every other one of which had come from the store.

Here's where it gets interesting. As I helped one of my daughters add items to her plate, one of the volunteers was asking kids what kind of dressing they wanted to dip veggies

---

[41] See exception number three: "The Birthday Party Rule."

in. Did they want ranch? Thousand island? Blue cheese? Then she came to my bottle, picked it up, and paused, eyeing it with suspicion.

"I don't know <u>what</u> this is," she said dismissively.

!!!

I know, right?

I could have pointed out that "this" was homemade, whereas all other options were store bought. I could have mentioned that "this" had four ingredients, whereas all other options had about forty. I could have mentioned that, of all the bottles on the table, "this" was the only one without any unpronounceable or unfamiliar ingredients, including stabilizers (diglycerides on your salad, anyone?), MSG (check your ranch!), or (need I even say it?) sugar.

But I didn't. Instead, I just felt keenly how topsy-turvy things have gotten when we are suspicious of foods for not being processed or manufactured *enough*.

Exhibit C: Candy-Based Summer Reading

When we got home from the festivities that afternoon, I literally poured our kids' backpacks out on the floor—papers, workbooks, projects, bottom of the desk dregs, and art class masterpieces were everywhere. Not to mention flyers advertising summer library programs, suggesting summer projects, and the Mother Myrick's Summer Reading Program Sheet...I saw that last one and my heart sank.

It sank because we've done the Mother Myrick's Reading Program for the last few years; Mother Myrick's is a nearby bakery and confectioner of some renown, and they offer special prizes to kids who bring in lists of the books they've been reading over the summer.

It's a great idea. It's also very generous. It's also a whole freakin' lot of candy. For every two books a kid reads, there is a corresponding little bag of candy and maybe some plastic toys or stickers. Last year, we actually made it to all five levels and Greta was up to her eyeballs in chocolate this and gummy that. It was a little overwhelming, but who was I to question the rules of the Summer Reading game?

However, this year I was the Sugar Nazi, and the Sugar Nazi questions bloody everything. I was in a bit of despair about having to sacrifice yet *one more* fun thing to the Gods of No Sugar, but I smiled and proposed an alternative to the kids: how about we make up our *own* Summer Reading Program? That was all they needed to hear—within minutes, Greta and Ilsa had found a large sheet of paper and were brainstorming prizes: How about berry picking? We could get a book at the bookstore…Swimming! No wait—bowling! Ooo! How about going to the *amusement park*!? They were giggling and squealing over the endless possibilities.

All at once I was relieved, impressed, and kind of humbled too. *Look at them go,* I thought. *They're taking on the challenge of retooling their world, their habits, their rewards system—they're excited about it!* We grown-ups, I think—so often stuck in our store-bought salad-dressing ruts—would do well to take a page from their book.

When school started up again in the fall, it was soon time for the sixth-grade overnight camping trip, which I had agreed to join Greta on. Immediately, I commenced worrying about the food situation.

Now, *could* I have brought my own food? Certainly after

everything we've learned this year I might've anticipated the upcoming sugar fest a mile away and packed a separate set of meals to bring. However, beside the not-insignificant issue of the bonding and group camaraderie (which, after all, was the point of the trip), there was a much more dire factor in my decision not to bring any food with me on the overnight: two of the girls in Greta's sixth-grade class have life-threatening food allergies. If I were to bring any food at all, I could have unwittingly posed a threat to these girls, way out in the Vermont wilderness. It was a nonissue; as far as I could tell, Deathly Allergies trump No-Sugar Experiments every time.

But that didn't mean we had to have dessert. No, sir. After months avoiding scores of sweets of every shape and size, I felt Greta and I were surely up to this paltry challenge. That was, of course, until I learned what that camping trip dessert was slated to be.

S'mores.

Oh *no!* I thought. Not...*s'mores!*

You see, when you're finished with this book, you will officially know all my Achilles' heels. A nice glass of red wine. A tiny but perfect little scoop of Italian gelato. Anything at all that combines chocolate and peanut butter. And, my goodness, that flamboyant love child of camping and convenience food, the s'more.

I have a deeply ingrained memory of my very first s'more: it was at sleep-away camp. I was eleven and desperately homesick. One night, we had a campfire in the center of our ring of canvas tents, and it was chilly and pitch dark. Since I was a s'more novice, a fellow camper showed me the proper technique for melting the chocolate rectangle on top of the graham cracker square by balancing them on a rock near the flames while you toasted your marshmallow on a stick. I scraped the hot marshmallow onto the ever-so-slightly melted chocolate with the help of the second half of the graham cracker and took a bite of what I suddenly realized was the single most delicious thing in the world.

Of course, I've had many, many s'mores since then (I insisted we have them the night of our wedding reception, for example), but none was ever as good as that very first one. Maybe it wasn't about the s'more as much as it was about everything else that night: the campfire, the after-dark chill in the air, the fact that I was away from home, *really* away, for the first time, and it being exhilarating and frightening and eye-opening all at the same time. I was beginning to realize that I could exist as a person without my family to lean back on, to define me, and decide for me what I thought. And my homesickness changed, evolved into a new kind of strength I had never known before.

Yes, all that can come from one good s'more memory.

So you see my dilemma. Granted, being my daughter means that Greta has had her share of s'mores from the get-go. ("Is that car engine over there on fire? Honey, where are the marshmallows?") And yet, could I bring myself to deny Greta what seemed to me to be a reasonable facsimile of my own s'more experience? Surrounded by her friends, far from home, on the verge of pre-adulthood? How much of a hypocrite *was* I?

And so, after a Hamlet-like hemming and hawing (To s'more? Or *not* to s'more?) I decided we would embrace the s'more. In the end, I was awfully glad we did—despite being really, truly, ridiculously sweet, they are still one of the most delicious things I can possibly imagine. The thing is, it only, *only* works if you are tired and sweaty, muddy and smoky, and sitting around a campfire in the dusk in the middle of nowhere. (Anywhere else? Not, repeat, NOT the same. My next bumper sticker will read: *Ban the Microwave S'more!*) Greta, for her part, was so giddy to enjoy the forbidden treat that she was dancing.

But it was more than that, more than just what our taste buds were telling us. We all, kids and parents alike, partook together of the same foods that night—capped off by the sensory fireworks display of the s'more—and I was reminded of that strange, ineffable bonding power in the sharing of food, even if it's just hamburgers and chips on plastic plates. I was glad of my decision to participate in the meals fully, for reasons on many levels.

As for *the rest* of the food, every item on the dinner menu that night had both a sugar and non-sugar option: Green salad (great!) with dressing (sugar!)? Hamburger or hot dog (fine) with ketchup (sugar!!)? Potato chips (okay) with BBQ flavor (sugar!!!)? If you picked and chose carefully, you could either avoid sugar almost entirely, or enjoy a meal overflowing with that nonessential ingredient we love so well. Amazing how easy it is to go from one extreme to another—how similar two plates could look even while one is loaded down with that familiar toxin and the other abstains. Because we knew what to choose, we got through dinner relatively unscathed.

Breakfast the next morning, however, made dinner look monastic by comparison. Breakfast was sugar with sugar and would you like some sugar on that? My head was reeling: hot cocoa (sugar) was followed by Nutri-Grain bars (sugar), graham crackers (sugar), and white bread (sugar) with jam (sugar). There was also a choice of banana or apple, which were the only sources of fructose (sugar) still at least wedded to their original fiber. All that was missing from this meal was whipped cream, sprinkles, and a cherry.

"But what *could* you have done?" you may well ask. Way out there in the middle of nowhere with no omelet station in sight? Well, we could've brought bagels, with hard-boiled eggs and cream cheese in our coolers. We could've made plain oatmeal over our campfire and washed it down with some cups of peppermint tea. Yes, as we have seen, breakfast—even a camping breakfast—is hard. But it's not impossible.

However, in this instance, we had no choice but to have dessert for breakfast and hope that somehow we would magically be able to create enough energy out of it to power us through the hour-long hike back out of the forest that was to follow. How do they expect these kids to function on a breakfast like this? I wondered, wide-eyed. I was horrified to recall that it was not all that different from what is served every day for the *school* breakfast.

Now, let me reiterate once more, for those who might have missed it previously, that I LOVE our school. I love our teachers, and I think they are incredible and amazing people for daring to lead this excursion of preteenagers into the woods every year—they certainly don't have to. They do it, I imagine, because they know it will be a terrific bonding experience for their students, that it will stay with them as a powerful memory not only throughout the school year, but—and I'm not overstating the matter here—throughout their entire lives. Small childhood events can have magical power like that.

Many of the kids on this trip had never been camping before. A significant number had never even *been* to the forest and farmland where it was held, despite the fact that we all live within a few miles of it and that its walking trails are free and open to the public. The kids were wildly excited about small things: telling scary stories around the campfire, getting to sleep sardine-style in the lean-to, playing Manhunt with flashlights in the dark, having s'mores.

So far be it from me to rain on the parade. The problem, as far as I can tell, *isn't* the teachers or really even the school as much as it is the culture that has grown accustomed to eating sugar with every meal and, frequently, in every item on our plates. This is what we have come to consider normal. How do you undo "normal"? That's the $64,000 question.

I got to know the kids in my daughter's grade better than ever before on the course of this overnight, and I have to tell you—they're fascinating. I was endlessly impressed by their humor and creativity and leadership and resilience and energy. But I'm deeply worried about them and what the future holds in store for them if we can't fix our food culture in time.

———

Interestingly, most people necessarily assumed going for a year without sugar would be harder on the kids than the grown-ups, and most of the time I shared that assumption.

Then every once in a while, my kids would surprise me. Like the morning I asked if Ilsa would like some bananas on her oatmeal. It was the kind of question we ask that is a total formality, in the vein of "Would you like to have an after-school snack?" or "Would you like to go on that roller coaster?"

But Ilsa stopped me in my tracks. "No," she said.

!

I was pretty sure I had misunderstood, so I asked her again. "No," she repeated. "Sometimes I like to have it without."

!!

Instead of asking her "Who are you and what have you done with my six-year-old?" I watched her eat an entire bowl of oatmeal with milk. Plain. And then, as if the forces of the universe hadn't toyed with my sense of the proper order of things quite enough, Greta came in next and proceeded to do the very same thing.

The thought suddenly occurred to me: perhaps children may have an easier time with the omission of sugar in their foods, since they haven't had as many years to get addicted as us tall people.

It wasn't the only time such a thing happened either. Once it started to get warm out, both kids had been mentioning that not having ice cream in summer was going to be one of the hardest parts of the project. Therefore, when I saw some plastic make-your-own-Popsicle molds, I jumped at the chance to replicate an ice-cream-ish experience in our own no-sugar universe.

———

I felt a lot better after I wrote to you about the ice cream problem. Because I didn't sleep that well because of that incident. Also I forgot to add that Kristina said that it was my choice because I was at school. Which she is right, but I'm trying to keep honest with the sugar diet. And that is at the best of my abilities. Well, got to go—Mom's making soft-boiled eggs & cantaloupe.

—from Greta's journal

———

Greta was especially excited and asked to make them…repeatedly. Folks, this child has the determination of a jackhammer.

After a few days of not making popsicles I, in desperation, ran out and bought the ingredient we had been lacking: yogurt. We raced home and mixed up a batch of banana yogurt popsicles that were—hooray!—frozen by dinner.

You know where I'm going with this: they loved them. The kit makes six popsicles, so we were set for a satisfying dessert for the next three nights. Next time around, I tried to be a bit more creative, adding in fresh strawberries so they turned pink in the blender (turning anything pink is always a good move in a house with two girls) and then adding some frozen berries to float randomly about like little prizes. Again—super big hit. Huge.

But here's the kicker: one night I tried one and—don't tell the kids, but—I wasn't as impressed as they were. It was good but…very icy. Like sucking on a milk icicle. And not, forgive me, *sweet* enough. *Gasp!*

So there you have it. I had officially become fussier than my kids. Imagine.

CHAPTER 10

MEET THE HERMITS

Originally, when I first contemplated the idea of a Year of No Sugar, images of cravings, temptation, and deprivation came to mind. My personal mental picture involved me in an Old West–style showdown with one of those wonderful square Ritter chocolate bars: "Let's go, *chocolate*," I'd sneer, perhaps from under a sombrero. "You and me. *Mano a mano*." You know, if chocolate had hands.

But in truth, what I was finding was that the hardest moments *weren't* solitary, quite the opposite. In fact, if I could just home-school the kids and avoid all restaurants and social events for the year—in other words, if we could just move to a new address under a convenient rock—the project would be a comparative snap. Turns out, at least for me, the social isolation of being on a different wavelength from the rest of the world around you was one of the most difficult parts of all.

For example, one day in April we attended the biggest local event I'd seen in my fourteen years in our town: a fundraiser to benefit the owners of a general store that had burned to the ground in the middle of the night two weeks prior. The event was so sudden, so shocking, so deeply upsetting to the community, that within hours plans were being fomented on Facebook for what would eventually blossom into a huge community expression of support and love: the resulting blow-out event featured a pig roast and chicken barbecue, a silent auction of over a hundred items, a bake sale of gargantuan proportions, live music by a local honky-tonk band, a swing set raffle, tractor rides, and face painting. Phew! We showed up at five minutes after two in the afternoon—as the event was scheduled to begin at two—to find hundreds and hundreds of people *already* in line for all of the above. But most of all, they were in line for the *food*.

Now, we'd been doing no sugar for months now, so you might think by this point I'd have figured this food thing out, right? But then there's that annoying fact that I can be—only *sometimes*, mind you—a little slow on the uptake. Honestly, amazingly, it really didn't *occur* to me that we wouldn't be able to eat the majority of food on the menu for this event until we were already there. Meat and pasta salad? Fine, right? Wait—no, pasta salad would have mayonnaise, the pork and chicken had barbecue sauce, so, um, what else? Baked beans, coleslaw…sugar was certainly in most of the menu items if not all of them. And you can't very well go to an event like this, with hundreds in line behind you waiting their turn, and start asking volunteers nit-picky questions about the pasta salad. You just *can't*.

Fortunately, we had been assuming we'd eat there later in the afternoon as an early dinner, and we *had* eaten lunch, so we weren't starving. Instead, we focused on everything else: we bought event T-shirts, we bid on items at the silent auction, the kids swung (swang?) on the raffle swing set and got their faces painted. Practically everyone in town made an appearance that afternoon, and in a town of just over a thousand people, that amounts to a great big party where you know virtually all of the guests. Now, in our neighborhood, a fundraiser is considered a walloping success if it raises anywhere near the thousand-dollar mark. At the end of this particular event an unheard-of $30,000 was raised to help store owners Will and Eric, who wandered around the event looking dazed by the outpouring of support.

Hi, it's 10:25 at night but still I faithfully write. Tonight my family and me went to a party. But part of it was fun, part of it was NOT. See, some people had brought sugar cookies and several kids were eating them in front of me. I bet they didn't mean to. And then "Norbert" (not his real name)...asked if we (me and Ben) wanted any candy. I said that I wouldn't like any and he said the same. Ben also said that it would rot our teeth...

So later I found out that Norbert was telling everyone that me and Ben had ruined it for everyone.

—from Greta's journal

Then friends of my two girls started appearing, licking soft-serve ice creams. Now *this* was hard. Reeeeeeally hard. You know how parents used to say "This hurts me more than it hurts you"? As a kid, you never believe it, but as a parent, you learn the true meaning of this. I would've given anything to hand them each a dollar and tell them to, of *course*, go get an ice cream. But. What kind of message would that have sent? How many more special events were to come this summer at which special exemptions would be begged? How many *more* times would we give in, and at what point would our project cease to have any real meaning?

So the afternoon progressed and we watched virtually the entirety of our town file through the line that snaked through the firehouse parking lot and all the way down to the road. I heard, at its peak, the wait for food was over an hour. But we never did join the line. We chatted with our neighbors. We checked our bids at the auction. We avoided the bake-sale table. We swung.

I came home with an empty feeling in me that only partly had to do with the fact that it was getting to be dinnertime. Everyone in the community had come together to help our neighbors Will and Eric, and we were a part of that, certainly. But we all know food is symbolic; food is important. When people break bread together, it means something. At least for the time being, our family was, in some small way, existing apart.

———————

The day *before* the event, like everybody else, we had gone to drop off our family's auction donation at the firehouse. It was very social, everyone standing around and marveling at the variety and quality of different auction items. ("Have you seen *this* one?") But what I really reeled at was on a table across the room: the bake-sale table. Goodies of every conceivable shape and size were crowded across two nine-foot tables, jostling for space, in the process of being neatly cataloged and labeled by my friend Rhonda. Rhonda was one of the event's organizers and also a reader of my blog, who regularly posted comments and links to interesting sugar-related articles she came across.

You read about torture. Like with verbal torture and killing torture. But I'm talking about a whole different kind of torture. And because of this Sugar thing, I had to experience it. It happened when Dutchie's—a local store—burned down (and) the people around near the store decided to give a benefit. So tomorrow is the benefit and we went to drop off some things we were donating to the silent auction and then we saw the bake sale. It had so many cakes, pastries, brownies and cookies it made my mouth water and my sister's too. It made me so mad to be on the sugar diet. It made so mad that I almost cried.

—from Greta's journal

Staring wide-eyed at the spread of frostings, sprinkles, chips, jellies, and coconut cream, I joked with Rhonda that I should take a photo of the awe-inspiring spread to post on my blog.

"Oh no!" she said, genuinely taken aback. "But…this is *good*!"

Her reaction stuck with me, because I think it has everything to do with how inextricably emotion and food are intertwined in our culture. I mean, of *course* it's good, right? The outpouring of emotion was physically visible in response to what was a shocking and violent event. People wanted to express love and comfort in the name of Will and Eric, to literally wrap them up in all that is warm and good and predictable, in an effort to make up for the scary thing that had changed their lives forever. What better way to do this than with a nice coffeecake or tray of raspberry thumbprints? We all understand, implicitly, when dessert is intended this way, as a concrete manifestation of love.

Similarly, another day Steve and I found ourselves at a potluck memorial service (yes, in Vermont we can make anything a potluck), and it struck me in very much the same way: one huge, long table of actual lunch food ran parallel to an equally long and huge table filled *entirely* with sweets—perhaps twenty feet by three of sugar, sugar, and more sugar. Again, should we be surprised if the outpouring of emotion naturally gravitated toward carrot cake and not carrots?

I'm not saying this is bad exactly, but Rhonda's reaction made me realize how deep and primal our attachment to sugar as love and comfort runs. I mean, of *course* raising money for a good cause is inherently a good thing. But when we lay out a football field of sugar in the name of comfort, I also think it's important to take a step back and think about the lesson we're teaching our children.

Because, after all, who's going to be eating a lot of those cookies and brownies, anyway?

What Rhonda's comment made me realize is that it's all well and good to demonize sugar when you're talking about the Big Bad Corporations sneaking high-fructose corn syrup into our ketchup and mayonnaise; it's another thing entirely to go after Grandma's lovingly baked molasses cookies. The problem is, nutritionally, your body can't tell the difference between the "bad" sugar (from Big Food Inc.) and "good" sugar (from Grandma). Fructose is fructose. And an excess of fructose consumption, now at its highest levels ever and still climbing, is making our society sick.

I imagine that one day, when the data has become so abundant as to be incontrovertible, having a buffet of sugar that rivals the actual food will be considered as socially unacceptable as smoking on airplanes or littering out your car window—things which we as a society once accepted as completely normal yet now we have come to realize the destructiveness of. Nobody is trying to say we can't smoke or drink or throw things away; they're just saying we have to be careful—*much* more careful—about how we go about it. Same with sugar.

Unfortunately, we seem to have a knack for being preoccupied with all the wrong messages. Remember when I was at the Mayo Clinic with my dad? One day we were eating lunch in the cafeteria when a rather heavyset couple sat down at the other end of our table. They had clearly gotten the "I'm trying to be good, or mostly good" meal; they each had purchased a large chef's salad with a breadstick, and she had added to her tray a banana and a skim milk, while he had a large diet soda and a piece of pie for dessert. I couldn't help but wonder to myself if they wouldn't have been better off enjoying a meal with much more fat but much less sugar/fake sugar. I mean, sugar (or the chemically fake stuff) was in the salad dressing, the breadstick, the diet soda, and in the pie. It was freakin' *everywhere* on their tray, and it was as if I—through some mutant power that might qualify me to be a comic book superhero—was the *only one who could see it*. I idly wondered if perhaps one of them suffered from one of the many variants of metabolic syndrome, and if so, if anyone would ever offer the suggestion that they might be healthier forgoing the salad with dressing in favor of the pot roast and mashed potatoes.

Heresy! Right?

Now, I've made it clear I'm no doctor, no nurse, and no dietitian. But it just makes a lot of *sense* to me when Dr. Robert Lustig says that we're effectively missing the Technicolor elephant in the living room when we caution people to watch their salt, watch their fat, watch their alcohol, but rarely if ever do we mention the deleterious effects of sugar and its omnipresence in our contemporary diet. Only veeeeeery recently have we seen sugar begin to become a part of the conversation, in part due to the efforts of people—Lustig, Gillespie—willing to say loudly and repeatedly what no one wants to hear. Another reason we may be willing, at last, to consider sugar's dark side is simply out of sheer desperation. It's beginning to seem like not a week goes by without another horrifying statistic being released about the obesity of Americans. Currently one quarter of young people in the United States now have diabetes or pre-diabetes! Seventeen percent of children and teenagers are now obese! By 2030 forty-two percent of all Americans will be obese! I know I'm repeating myself, but it's hard to imagine worse statistics than these.

So maybe, just maybe, if enough of us pester our poor waitresses for ingredients and start reading the depressing labels on the foods in our supermarket, just *maybe* the momentum will stick and the dialogue will at last start to change. Very early on in our Year of No Sugar, my mother sent me a short newspaper article in which it was noted that the "just-released...Dietary Guidelines say that we should 'significantly reduce' our intake of added sugars..."

"That's because diets high in added sugar are linked not only to obesity, but also to an increased risk of high blood pressure, triglycerides, inflammation, and low levels of good HDL cholesterol."[42]

---

[42]Molly Kimball, "Secret Sweets," *The Times Picayune*, February 11, 2011.

Yes! Thank you! Not only that, then the article goes on to list all the products you'd never suspect to find sugar in such as salad dressing, ketchup, bagels, pasta sauce, and bread. Sound familiar? Of course, as we now know, if she had wanted to, the author could've added exponentially to her list: chicken broth, mayonnaise, breakfast cereal, dried fruit, English muffins, baby food, pita bread, coleslaw, virtually every sauce known to man…She really should've given me a call.

That's okay. The article was tiny, but I was impressed that it existed at all. Some time after that, Gary Taubes wrote the extensive article "Is Sugar Toxic?" for the *New York Times Magazine*. And after that HBO released a four-part documentary on obesity in America titled *Weight of the Nation*. And a little while after that, Mayor Bloomberg banned the bucket soda in New York City.[43] I wondered, could it be that we might be just beginning to have a revelation that reverses so much of what we've been told about nutrition for so long?

In his YouTube lecture, Lustig had stated it as plain as can be: "It's not the fat, people. *It's not the fat.*"

I wished, somehow, I could have communicated that to our table mates at Mayo Clinic that day and saved them from who knows how many bad salads, not to mention a lifetime of trying to be "good" and wondering why it still isn't working.

---

[43]Despite the fact that this measure was subsequently struck down by the State Supreme Court (March 2013), I still adore Bloomberg for this. Whether it was legally correct or not, I love the fact that he stuck his own political neck out in order to get us debating the horse-trough-size soda cup.

CHAPTER 11

WHY AM I NOT ITALIAN?

One day I woke up and realized that we had made it to a significant milestone: we were officially past the six-month mark. Halfway!! Could it be that we had really made it so far? Could it really be that we had so much farther to go? June had been clammy and wet, so by the time July rolled around, most area residents were figuring summer had simply decided not to come this year. This is Vermont; it happens. But just as I was waking up to realize our No-Sugar Year was halfway to its finish line, I was also waking up to realize that summer really was going to arrive after all. All of a sudden the marble quarry–swimming hole was full of people showing off their farmer tans. Before I had fully realized it had started, strawberry season was practically over, so I hurried out and bought two quarts, never mind going picking.

Yes, summer had finally arrived, just in time for us to go away. We were preparing for a trip—a big trip. We would be leaving in a few days for two weeks in Italy.[44]

---

[44] This would be our second visit to Italy as a family—the first was that trip when Greta missed the third-grade lesson on fractions.

Now I know what you're thinking. You're *not* thinking, *Gee, did Eve's family visit the Leaning Tower of Pisa? The Vatican? The Coliseum?* I know you're not thinking that because that's not what everyone at home was asking me. What everyone at home was asking me was: "Oo! *What* are you going to do about the Sugar Project?"

Yeeeaaaaah. Good question. It was one to which I had given much thought but had yet to receive any brilliant revelations about. At the time, my circular thought pattern ran something like this: the Italians are serious about their food—in particular fresh, homemade food; this will be extremely helpful.[45] Also very helpful will be the fact that the Italians aren't too big on desserts—gelato and tiramisu notwithstanding. The first time our family went to Italy two years before, I recall more than one instance in restaurants when we had to ask if, in fact, there *was* any dessert to be had. We were much more likely to be offered an after-dinner drink of limoncello or amaro than a dessert menu. It was often an afterthought, as in: "Oh! Yeah—sure we have dessert! *Would* you like dessert?"

On that trip, the desserts we did order struck my American palate as...not very good. Instead, they were creamy and cakey and lemony and almondy. They were not what I would call...*sweet*. I didn't care for them very much—at that time, I was still looking for that taste explosion at the end of a good meal to signify its end, like fireworks at the end of the Fourth

---

[45] In fact, the Slow Food Movement began in Italy—did you know that? Legend has it that in 1986, it began as a protest against a McDonald's slated to open at the foot of the Spanish Steps. And in fact, I've *been* to that McDonald's with my kids, which is to say, we used their convenient public restroom.

of July. I mean, you just can't go *home* till the grand finale practically blows your eardrums out—or taste buds off as the case may be. We Americans are not big on subtlety.

Therefore, by comparison, my logic went, we should be in good shape, right? No one would be tempting us with deep-fried Oreos or Death-by-Chocolate Sundaes.

However, gelato is good. Really, *really* good. Did you know that you can sometimes request *crema* and they will put a perfect, tiny little dollop of whipped cream on top of your gelato cone? Did you know it was projected to be between eighty and ninety degrees the entire first week of our trip? Do you think, at the tourist-thronged landmarks we were sure to be visiting, we were going to be encountering gelato every blinking where we went?

This, I realized, was going to present a problem. If we had any hope of surviving the trip with our No-Sugar Project intact, Steve and I needed to come up with our Official Italian Strategy.

So one night when we had a babysitter, Steve and I hashed it out over dinner.

My husband started out the bargaining. "How about one dessert per day?" he helpfully suggested. I about spit out my drink. I pointed out that, on a fourteen-day trip, this would result in us having more desserts in the month of *July* than we would otherwise have in the entirety of our yearlong project.

"How about one dessert for the whole trip—our July dessert?" I countered. The look of abject horror on his face was impressive.

"Now, we're not going halfway around the world to torture our children with wonderful ice cream they can't have." Oo! The "torturing your children" card. Well played!

"How about one dessert per week?" I re-countered. As you can imagine, this haggling would go on to consume a good portion of our evening.

———————

Here's what Mom does with the rules. Makes them.
—from Greta's journal

———————

Other ideas were floated: what about family voting on a case-by-case basis? Although this appealed to my democratic side, I'm reasonably confident that my otherwise very supportive family, when faced with an Italian gelato stand in all its glory, would nonetheless vote the No-Sugar Project out every time—quite possibly before breakfast.

By the end of our meal, we seemed to have reached some sort of loose consensus: we would, of course, have our July dessert in Italy. Very likely, (I hated to admit) we would end up having more than one dessert during the course of our trip. Whatever we had would have to be rare and special. So, basically, we were going to wing it.

On the whole, Italians seem to have gotten the sweets question right—enjoying little, wonderful, golf-ball-size scoops of gelato as a special treat is a lesson we "more-is-more" Americans would do well to learn. Then again, I've been to Italy four times in my life, and every time I've gone, I've been dismayed to see that the gelato scoops have gotten a little bit bigger. Ever so gradually, they're becoming more and more American. Sigh.

I wish it wouldn't. I adore Italy. I adore it just as it is, no Americanization necessary, thank you. I hate when we enter a restaurant and they hand us the English menus; I hate that they *have* English menus. I love that my children have eaten wild boar and roasted rabbit in Italy. Why have they done this? In part, it's because the Italians have no concept of the children's menu, which is a wonderful, wonderful thing. The day I go to a sit-down restaurant in Italy and my children can order chicken nuggets with fries is the day I stop going to Italy.

Not only had I been lucky enough to have visited Italy before, but my first trip there had been when I spent an entire college semester in Rome studying art and architecture. That entire four-month period was a frenetic time—every weekend all the students rose at four or five a.m. to board an air-conditioned bus that carted us through a dizzying array of hill towns, Etruscan ruins, and crazy modern architecture. We often stopped in a given town only long enough to visit the church or the museum or the postmodern cemetery, reboard the bus, and move on. It must have seemed to the residents like an invasion of ravenous sheep: the professors leading the flock of us, sketching and photographing everything in sight. We were young; we were American; we were stupid. As we peered over the edges of our sketchbooks, we were easily confused. "Was that Gubbio?" "No, that was Assisi." "I thought it was Orvieto…"

During that far-off time, we had done a drive-by visit of Florence in which I was able to see almost nothing—it was Sunday and raining, and all the museums had been closed. Ever since, I had longed to go back and see what it was I had missed—the Uffizi, the Pitti Palace, the Duomo…heck, Michelangelo *himself* was calling me, gently reprimanding me for having neglected *la bella citta* for far too long.

And thus, at long last, following the red-eye flight, I

arrived in Florence with my family bright and early one July morning, in a state of exhaustion that can only be described as hallucinatory. Within a day, we had mostly recovered and were fully immersed in Florence: our ancient apartment, the Ponte Vecchio just down the hill, the mazelike supermarket where you had to bring your own bags or risk having the counter girl roll her eyes at the ridiculous Americans. And it was *hot*—sweat running down the back of your legs hot—so every afternoon we returned to our little hole in the wall to sleep off the heat and the bottle of wine we had consumed with our incredible lunch. Almost overnight, we all felt we had been transported to another life and that we had left America far, far behind.

In some ways, it felt like we'd left the No-Sugar Project at home too. This is not to say we weren't *doing* No Sugar—we were. It just seemed to…*matter* less. We went through entire meals, entire *days* worth of meals, enjoying incredible tastes—freshly made al dente pasta; thinly sliced, delicately salty prosciutto; crunchy, garlic-rubbed crostini with pungent green olive oil—all without having to ever give much thought to The Sugar Problem. As long as we ignored the small table of *dolci* we passed by on our way to find the restroom, we found ourselves getting along for long stretches of time without the thought even occurring to us that we were missing something.

Okay, I must admit I wasn't being the Spanish Inquisition there the way I had been at home—but by the same token, I didn't have to be. Did I actually *ask* if there is sugar in the freshly made *pici*? No, but I already know the ingredients of *pici*: flour and water. Do I need to *ask* the ingredients of things like *prosciutto e melone* or *insalata Caprese* (tomatoes, basil leaves, and mozzarella)? It would be like asking what the ingredients are in my morning eggs or my glass of water.

So what's up with that anyway? Italians have believed in fresh and local foods long before anyone ever dreamed up the term *locavore*. When I lived in Rome as a student, I had been amazed to attend the morning markets and find produce so fresh it still had dew and little bits of dirt on it. It took me a while to get used to the idea of going to so many different places just to compose a meal: the outdoor market for fruits and vegetables, the butcher for meat,[46] the bakery for fresh bread and pasta. But after a while, the genius behind it made sense—get the foods from the people who are the experts in them, spend the extra time because, really, what could *be* more important? What, you have something *better* to do? Like what?

Unlike us ever-trendy Americans, Italians' belief in such things doesn't strike me as stemming from a desire to save the planet or preserve the polar bears or even to benefit their own health. No, food comes close to being a second religion there for the deceptively simple reason that *they know what's good*.

I got that phrase from my grandmother, who used to use it to approvingly describe someone who knew how to appreciate something important, usually food. Scratch that—*always* food. As in, "Of *course* he likes the schnitzel! *He* knows what's good." Even though she was of German heritage, not Italian, the sentiment was exactly the same: *what* could be more important than really, *really* good food?

Don't get me wrong. It's not like sugar had suddenly

---

[46]As a vegetarian-of-some-kind-or-other at that time, I skipped the trip to the butcher.

disappeared. We were having our share of sugar thrown at us on this trip, just not in the restaurants. On the two Swiss Air flights it took to get there, the flight attendants kept trying to hand us Swiss chocolate bars—and how often do you really think people say no to those? We arrived—at looooong last on nooooo sleep—to the apartment we had rented to find a huge dish of hard candies on the coffee table, little wrapped *Baci* thoughtfully placed by the bedside, and a huge tub of complimentary tiramisu ice cream in the freezer—specifically *per le bambine*, our landlord explained.

Need I mention the entire supermarket rows of nothing but four million kinds of snack cookies? The fact that they have approximately three gelato stands for every one tourist? (It's as if the people from Planet Gelato invaded years ago and no one noticed.) Sure, Europeans like their Cokes and their Nutella as much as anyone else. You can't say they don't have a sweet tooth, just that sweets aren't so *insidious* there as in American culture. What I noticed most of all was that it was a fairly easy separation if it's something you want to separate.

And crazy us, we wanted to. Though some days I was trying hard to remember why...

Now, before I go any farther I'd just like to state, for the record, that I'm really, really lucky. I know. I have two incredible daughters who *like food*. REAL food, things like calamari and miso soup. Greta likes to brag about having eaten snails in Paris and is impatient with the kids' menu at most restaurants, choosing instead a flank steak or penne alla vodka from the adult menu. Ilsa is, if anything, even more enthusiastic: in Italy we could order her a cheese plate or a *crostini misti*—which includes chicken liver paté—and she'd be happy as a clam in butter.

Sometimes, when I forget how lucky we really are, I'll be reminded by the apprehensive look of a waiter or dining companion who will cautiously ask, "Do you think they will...?"

"Eat that? Sure!" I'll respond without thinking. Later, I realize what they were *really* asking: "Will your child melt down if anything other than mac 'n' cheese or pasta with butter fails to appear at their place setting?"

I'd love to take credit for all this culinary open-mindedness, but honestly, I'm not sure: are fussy eaters born or made?

Of the two, Ilsa might be the one most interested in food, possibly because she is always hungry. She's the child who takes twice as long as everyone else at the table to finish her dinner, and then five minutes after the plates have been cleared asks if there's anything to eat. Frequently, she will ask when lunch is, entirely unaware that we've already eaten it. The ongoing Ilsa refrain is "Mommy, I'm still hungry. Do you have any food in your purse?" And because I'm Ilsa's mom, I always do.[47]

This combination of appetite and willingness to try new things came in handy the night we went to the Teatro del Sale in Florence—an absolute high point of our trip. It had been highly recommended to us by a very gracious local, and she assured us that it would be fine for the kids as well. All we knew was that it involved dinner and a show of some sort, we should call to reserve our places, and go early in order

---

[47]During our No-Sugar Year, this meant I carried a lot of Larabars, the ones that are composed entirely of nuts and dried fruit: Apple Pie, Lemon, and Peanut Butter being our favorites. Of course nuts and unsweetened dried fruit always worked for portable snacks, as did the Super Cookies by the brand GoRaw, which have three ingredients: coconut, sesame seeds, and dates.

to "join"…whatever *that* meant. I was nervous what we were getting ourselves into. Me being the only one who could speak any Italian in our family, I felt it was all on my shoulders whether we had an exciting, truly "Italian" evening or ended up embarrassing ourselves in some uniquely "We're not from here!" way. Would we get fed? Would there be some terribly inappropriate show? Would we even *find* the place? But my curiosity was too great; we *had* to try.

We arrived at 7:30 on the dot, dressed up and out of breath from hurriedly walking several blocks in this unfamiliar part of town, nestled in the labyrinth of residential streets that spiral off from the historic Centro. After some confusion, I ascertained in my mishmash Italian that we each had to fill out forms—the kids too—and pay a small fee to "join" the "cultural circle." Once this was accomplished, we were given gorgeous membership cards that put my Vermont driver's license to shame and we stumbled inside, where we could now pay for our evening's attendance at…whatever this was.

It wasn't cheap—at thirty euro per person, I fervently hoped this included everything. I learned it did, once the helpful man at the cash register began speaking English unprompted in order to be sure we understood the way the evening would work. Oh well, so much for my flawless Italian.

It would be a buffet, he described. VERY long. There would be, as he put it, "surprises." Wine and water were self-serve by carafes in the lobby, and please, he cautioned, take it easy. I wondered if the emphasis on pacing ourselves over the course of a "VERY long" meal was because we had small children or because we were Americans. And I was a little apprehensive. I mean, how long was *long*?

Turns out, *long* is about two hours. Heck—practically

every Italian meal we ever *had* took about that long. I could see, however, that it would be easy to go overboard in an atmosphere such as this one. At the far end of the room there was a buffet table featuring a battalion of help-yourself casseroles, salads, and breads; couscous, hummus, warm potato salad, lentils, shiny beets. Just when we thought we had amassed plenty of food on our plates and found seats, suddenly a man's head appeared in the window of a glass wall that showcased the kitchen—a Willy Wonka's factory of delicious handmade delicacies where all *kinds* of things seemed to be going on—and he began to bellow as if announcing the contenders in an important boxing match. ("*And in this cor-NAH!*") Although I never managed to catch it all, it became clear that every few minutes he was heralding the presentation of a new dish, and that if you wanted to try some, now was the time to sidle up to the window and receive a bread-plate-size portion of it.

The girls caught on very quickly to this arrangement and soon it was hard to keep them from popping up and down like little Jack-in-the-boxes. We tried nearly everything as the tiny courses rolled out one by one: chicken meatballs, fish soup, tiny clams in spicy broth, roast chicken and potatoes, tubular pasta with meat sauce...As advised, we tried to pace ourselves, but the girls were in heaven, particularly Ilsa.

"When's he gonna yell again?" she kept asking.

"These are so yummy, I just can't stop eating them!" she proclaimed about the mussels dressed with lemon juice, garlic, and olive oil.

"If this is still here when I grow up, I might want to work here," she said later, adding, "I could eat all the leftovers after!" At another moment, she explained that she was sure to return to Florence someday. "I would come here so I could eat this yummy food!"

I sat back and marveled at my children. How many six-year-olds, I wondered, would have felt similarly after being served unshelled shrimp so tiny and leggy they looked like large bugs? Certainly, we weren't the only tourists in the room—we heard a fair amount of English as we traipsed back and forth to bring our used plates to the dish window (another custom here) but ours were the only children.

At last, it was time to round out this fantastic culinary parade. Greta returned from her four-dozenth trip to the kitchen window to report that they were serving ice-cold glasses of dessert.

"It's...peach gelato," she said tentatively, avoiding my eyes.

"And we are going to have it!" I added with enthusiasm. Greta's and Ilsa's faces lit up like they had been plugged in. Looking back, this was the best decision I made on the trip; as far as I'm concerned, everything else could have fallen away—but for that one joyful evening, magical meal, and sweet, perfect, peach gelato.

After that, there was still more in store for us. The tables, which had seated perhaps one hundred "cultural circle" members, were whisked away and the room was filled with the sounds of scraping chairs and multilingual chatting as our dining room transformed into a performance hall, facing a modest stage at the far end of the room. We learned that the show tonight would be a Cuban trio accompanied by dancers.

For me, it was all like a very, very happy dream. As I sat there in the audience, wonderfully full of perfect bites of food and gulps of red wine, deeply breathing in the robust strains of guitar, I had one of those heartbreakingly rare moments when you feel that something has gone, somehow, incredibly, inexplicably, perfectly right.

Sometime later, Ilsa made one more comment to me on the topic of travel. "It's just that food around the world is *so good!*" she exclaimed.

I couldn't have said it better myself.

Later, on the plane coming home, I had a major attack of ambivalence. How had it *really* gone? Had we passed the No-Sugar tests reasonably enough or failed miserably? On the one hand, you *could* say we did pretty well. We drank cappuccino while everyone around us had gelato. We drank water, water, and more water. When, during the second half of the trip, we met up with relatives in northern Italy, they were kind enough to make special requests for us at restaurants and to engineer no-sugar versions of things like barbecue sauce for us when we ate in. We held fast to our individual exceptions and steered clear of so many fun European treats we would've *loved* to have: Nutella, flavored yogurts, those funny little snack cookies that Europeans do so well. We looked the other way repeatedly when passing elaborate shop windows filled with pyramids of chocolate truffles, fancy meringues, and exotic-looking candies.

And, as I mentioned before, sugar is infinitely easier to separate out in a place like Italy, easier to spot than in America, where its presence is so much more insidious and pervasive. It's true that ordering water instead of soda is actually considered a respectable option in Europe, whereas in America it's somehow slightly looked down upon as slightly odd or cheap. ("Oh, you're *just* having *water?*") And sure, I was well supplied with my big bag of Snacks For Emergencies, including coconut cookies and any fruit we managed to pick up along the way. Not to mention that we guiltily threw away more sugar than I care to think about—those complimentary Swiss chocolate bars, those chocolate *Baci*, and that tub of tiramisu ice cream.

And yet…

Like some sort of mutant slime from a cheesy horror movie, I kept feeling sugar creeping *back in*…around the ancient marble doorframes and through the windows' bulky wooden shutters, following us like shadows along the tourist-jammed streets. Small things, mostly. Once, Steve accidentally came home from the supermarket with a large vanilla yogurt rather than plain. Once, while staying the night in a B&B, I put granola on my plain yogurt in desperation to avoid the Nutella and sweet yellow cake that constituted the other breakfast options, all the while looking the other way while my kids ate cornflakes. (*Cornflakes*! Horrors!) Once, in a cafeteria across the street from Florence's famed Duomo, we picked out what we *thought* were strawberries and plain yogurts for the girls' snack, only to discover all that white stuff was *whipped cream*, not yogurt. Once, while having our unsweetened cappuccinos for a snack, we were sufficiently crazed with peckishness that we ate the hard little gingerbread cookies that had thoughtfully been placed on the saucers. Yes, these were the things keeping me up at night: whipped cream ambushes and postage stamp–size complimentary cookies.

Then again, other transgressions were bigger. Twice, our whole family succumbed to the siren song of gelato (only once, in my opinion, was worth it: that heavenly peach at the Teatro del Sale, with teeny little bits of skin throughout).

With an average of ninety-five degrees each day in Florence, and an average of fourteen tourists slurping a cone for every ten you passed on the street, keeping it to *only* twice was a Herculean effort along the lines of Superman reversing time.

Once, I heard our affable waitress describe the tiramisu as "*buonissima*" and I—swept away by the joy of a delicious meal and the fact that I was understanding far more of the Italian conversation than I had expected to—impulsively ordered two for the family to share…only to have it *not* be all that *buonissima* after all. Phoo.

Once, the girls and I partook of thin slivers of a delicious *crostata cioccolato* which was the birthday dessert of our eight-year-old cousin whose family we had met up with. This I justified as an implementation of the birthday party rule, which made sense except that it wasn't supposed to include *me*. Ahem.

This was the Dolomites, an alpine region of Italy so far to the north that prior to World War One it had been part of Austria…and, as it turns out, also a very dangerous place in which to send my husband off to the bakery. The first time he stumbled inadvertently upon the bakery, as if in a trance, wafted in on the scent of a fresh apple strudel, which he promptly bought—helplessly—only to then give it away to the relatives we had met up with. The second time he came home with a combination of sweet and savory pastries—speaking neither German nor Italian was a plausible excuse for his ingredient ignorance. But by the *third* time—when he was arriving home with little marzipan hedgehogs and delicately wrapped bars of chocolate embedded with animal crackers or hazelnuts—I knew we had to get out of there, *quick*.

Nonetheless, it is worth noting that none of these "sweet"

treats, when tried, yielded that sugar blast Americans are so fond of…While an apple strudel or chocolate pie in the United States wouldn't be considered worth its salt if it failed to make your teeth ache, the things we tried in bites here and there truly surprised us: apple strudel actually tasted like… *apples*; the birthday chocolate pie tasted of pastry and cream. No explosion of sweet; no King Kong–size portions. When we saw a Ben & Jerry's in Florence, I smiled ruefully and wondered what the Italians thought of ice cream flavors like Chocolate Chip Cookie Dough and Phish Food (which has marshmallow, caramel, *and* fudge in it) when juxtaposed with the elegant subtlety of, say, a lovely peach gelato. Do they think we've completely lost our minds? And are they right?

Back in Florence, on the last night, after very kindly being served complimentary biscotti as we tried to pay the dinner bill (help!), Steve and the girls had a good-bye treat of yet another gelato (that's three, for those keeping score) while I abstained. By that time, I could feel the ground moving beneath me. I agonized as I packed my suitcase. We had had *so* much more sugar here than we would have at home, yet *so* very much less than we would have had if not for The Project. What did that *mean*? Had we been good? Or *not* so good?

Both, I imagine. In fact, I suppose the answer was that we were human.

Once we returned home from our travels, I was happy to notice that my kids were more interested than ever in *food*: in ingredients, in the garden, in recipes and improvisation. The fact is, my kids were insisting to be let into the other side of the equation: they wanted to *cook*…and they were not taking no for an answer. This is great, right? In theory. But in practice, you get into things like sharp knives, hot stoves, and the fact that Mommy can't supervise right now because if she doesn't get some laundry done you'll both be going to school tomorrow in bathing suits. Kids cooking is wonderful if not always terribly convenient.

———

Kale Chips
  Cut down the middle of leaf of either side of the stem.
  Put the leaves in a bowl and coat the leaves in olive oil.
  Lay the leaves on either a baking sheet or parchment paper.
  300 bake for 10–15 minutes.
                                    —*from Greta's journal*

———

And also, if I'm entirely honest with myself, there's the fact that I often enjoy cooking alone—the peaceful meditation of chopping, kneading, mixing, and preparing has become a quiet pleasure I look forward to when I'm not in a frantic rush to produce sustenance NOW. It's not unusual for me to plan a more complicated meal some afternoon when I know I'll have a few hours to spend pulling it together and to look forward to it as me time. This had become even more the case since beginning the No-Sugar Project—as if to compensate for the lack of sweets, I seemed to focus more and more on the homemade, which may be simple but is definitely not always expedient.

Fresh pasta is a quintessential example. What could be more delicious? What could be simpler? What could be more of a pain in the tuchus? Inspired by our recent trip, I had been wanting to find an afternoon to make fresh gnocchi, which I learned to make a few years ago and have only attempted here at home a handful of times. (By the time I forget the consequent mountain of dishes and the several hours of work, it's usually about time for me to attempt it again.)

This time was different, however; this time the kids wanted to help. *Demanded* to help, actually. It was one of the last few summer days before school began again and I was savoring the luxury of spending the afternoon with them with no place to rush off to—no soccer practice, no ballet class, no library board meeting. And yet I felt conflicted...What if they screwed the pasta up? What if hours of work resulted in a gloppy, unpalatable mess? Then—panic attack—*what would we have for dinner*? (Remember, between living in the country and being on The Sugar Project, there weren't very many quick-fix options open to us when dinner goes suddenly, horribly wrong.) Now, there are times when me being such a relentless control freak has its benefits—this was not one of them.

I took a few deep breaths and decided to get over it. If we're going to teach our kids about real food, we are going to have to let them learn how to make it, now aren't we? I knew it was time to put my money where my mouth was.

Boy, I'm glad I did. They were amazing! In fact, after making the dough—kneading together fresh boiled potatoes, flour, and egg—the kids did all the work while I sat back and watched. And this is not an inconsiderable amount of work, either. Greta carefully sliced bits of dough from the large dough "loaf," rolling each one out into a long, quarter-inch diameter snake. Ilsa would take over at this point, cutting dozens of tiny gnocchi from the snakes the size of Tootsie Rolls; each tiny island of dough carefully kept separate on the cutting board so as not to have the pasta bits stick together. This was not Kraft Easy Mac. This took a *long* time. I was amazed at their tenacity, their patience.

Did everything go perfectly? No. At one point, in what will hereafter be referred to as the Great Gnocchi Massacre of 2011, Ilsa accidentally knocked the wooden cutting board— filled with little cut-up gnocchi—just off the counter enough to dump a good three dozen onto the kitchen floor. The three of us gasped. We were hushed for a moment, staring at the floor and thinking about the hard work that—*poof!*—was gone just like that. Then Ilsa ran off in tears.

Now, some people have a Little Devil on their shoulder. I have a Little Control Freak. The Little Control Freak whispered in my ear "See? Told you so. All that work. What will you have for dinner *now?*" Fortunately, I listened instead to the Mom Angel on my other shoulder who said, "There's still plenty of pasta left. Nobody died. It's fine." And of course, it really was. Soon, I managed to convince Ilsa of that fact as well, and we were back to the pasta factory.

In fact, it was better than fine. We had a lovely dinner that took us all afternoon to make and, boy, were the girls proud! And it was delicious—even if they weren't as ridiculously careful about it as I would have been. I mean, it's just potatoes, egg, and flour, right? Real, homemade food is desperately important—to our health, to animal welfare, to the environment—but fortunately for us, most of the time it's not rocket science. It just takes a little time. And patience.

CHAPTER 12

DESERT ISLAND DESSERTS

After the roller coaster of trying to keep everyone on the No-Sugar bandwagon in Italy (It's easy! It's hard!), it was lovely to return to the relative safety and comfort of home with our steadfast and simple rule: one dessert per month.

There will be those who will balk at this, I know, and perhaps with justification. "*How* can you have a Year of No Sugar *with* sugar?" they will ask. "How can you justify even one dessert per month? Does this *truly* count as a No-Sugar Year then?"

As I've mentioned, we're a *fairly* normal family. If this yearlong project had been a snap, then that would have been an entirely different book. (Maybe even a very short book: "We didn't eat any sugar. It was easy. The end.") I knew I'd never keep my hungry family of four on board a project of this magnitude without something, *something* to look forward to. "Don't worry, honey, you can have a birthday cake *next* year!" simply wasn't going to cut it, and for all my sugar bashing, I wasn't ready to do that to my kids as a parent, either. None of us was at all sure we could truly make it through this year, but if we knew we had just one special treat we could look forward to every other fortnight, it might just make the difference between success and giving up entirely.

Also, I was intrigued. I wanted to get back to a time, not so very long ago, when having dessert indicated a truly special occasion. As the story goes, the hot fudge sundae was so named because you could only order it on *Sunday*. (What? You mean, I can't have it on a Tuesday at 2 a.m.? How un-American is *that*?)

Of course, as it turned out, there was the aforementioned yet unforeseen benefit of the "sugar check-in" to see how our tongues and the rest of our bodies' reactions to fructose were changing over time. That turned out to be an intriguing saga in and of itself.

And lastly, I was just plain curious: what *would* we choose if we could only have twelve desserts in a year? What would be the best of the best? The desserts you'd want to take with you to that proverbial dessert island? The things *worth*, you know, consuming a little poison for?

Once a month we get a treat. To many people this is astonishing.

—from Greta's journal

It's interesting to see how the dessert parade played out— much differently, I think, than if we had sat down and planned it all in advance. Knowing me, I would have attempted a fairer cross-section of the dessert spectrum and would certainly not have allowed such a preponderance of pies, for example.

Then again, we did manage to get at least one instance of

THE OFFICIAL DESERT ISLAND DESSERTS

JANUARY: (Ilsa's Birthday) Ilsa's-Turning-Six Chocolate Cupcakes

FEBRUARY: (Valentine's Day) Not-Quite-For-Valentine's Chocolate Mousse

MARCH: Oh-My-God Sour Cherry Pie

APRIL: (Greta's Birthday) Great-Grandma's Sour Milk Chocolate Cake

MAY: Eve's-Childhood Rhubarb Pie

JUNE: (Father's Day) A&W Root Beer Floats

JULY: (Italy) Well-We're-Going-To-Say-Peach Gelato

AUGUST: Mister John's Mardi Gras Birthday Cake

SEPTEMBER: (Steve's Birthday) By Special-Request Emeril's Banana Cream Pie

OCTOBER: (Eve's Birthday) Peanut Butter Pie

NOVEMBER: (Thanksgiving) Pumpkin Pie with homemade whipped cream

DECEMBER: (Christmas) Grandma Sharon's Best-Ever Christmas Cookies

several different dessert types. In addition to the usual suspects of cake and pie, there were cookies, pudding (chocolate mousse), and ice cream (peach gelato), and even a dessert beverage in the form of the root beer float. We never repeated a dessert (except that technically, the Turning-Six Chocolate Cupcakes and the Sour Milk Chocolate Cake were made from the same basic cake recipe), and everyone got to pick a dessert *all by themselves* at least once.

Nine of the desserts were homemade, seven of which were made by me. My friend Katrina, horrified at the thought I might make my own birthday dessert, very generously made the peanut butter pie for me, and who better to make Grandma Sharon's Christmas cookies than Grandma Sharon? This left only three desserts that were store bought, representing a spectrum of sources: root beer floats from a fast food purveyor (horrors!), peach gelato from a restaurant, and the Mardi Gras birthday cake from a bakery. I feel like it's about time to make up a bar graph and calculate some percentages, but I'll attempt to restrain myself.

Instead, here are a few Monthly Treat Highlights:

January

Certainly, I was the most apprehensive about the *first* month's dessert, not just because it was the very first one, but more importantly because it was Ilsa's birthday in January, and I was pretty sure I'd never forgive myself if I screwed up something as important as my six-year-old's birthday cake. She's not going to turn six *again*, you know!

But really, what was there to mess up? I mean, Ilsa gets to pick the dessert—that one, special, once-per-month deal—I make it, everyone eats it, end of story! What's so nerve-wracking about *that*? Here was my problem—what we'd traditionally done for kid birthdays in our house is to have *two* celebratory desserts: one for the family party on the actual "real" birthday, followed by the "kids'" dessert at the kids' party that inevitably followed on a weekend.

Mind you, we don't even get *into* bringing cupcakes in for the class at school…nor do we put candy in goody bags for party guests to bring home. And then there's the fact that one can go to a kid's birthday party and have a meal consisting of pizza with sugar in the crust, sugar in the tomato sauce, and a big glass of sugar to drink, by which I mean fruit juice. By the time we get to the overt sugar of dessert, we parents often don't realize how much sugar they've *already had*. To sum up? Kids' birthday parties = sugar minefield.

But back to my problem: what *were* we going to do? Here we were, just beginning our project, on the veritable cusp of our No-Sugar Year, and already I was feeling pressure to compromise in the name of Not Being a Crappy Mom. Because this was only *two weeks* into the project, I had yet to conduct my infamous date-cookie experiments yet. I had yet to discover David Gillespie's recipe website or the wonders of dextrose. We *couldn't* have two January desserts, and we couldn't *not* serve dessert at the kids' party, so *what* were we going to have on Ilsa's actual sixth birthday? Unsweetened applesauce? Wouldn't the candles sink?

Then I had an idea. We would capitalize on the one No-Sugar dessert we had in our arsenal at that early point: frozen banana ice cream.

Following our traditional birthday meal of English muffin pizzas (after digging up alternative, no-sugar brands of English muffins and marinara sauce, of course) paired with some sautéed spinach, we stuck a candle in what I fervently hoped would be a delicious grand finale: banana splits: bananas halved, banana ice cream, topped with strawberries soaked in balsamic vinegar, whipped cream (minus the called-for sugar), and a fresh cherry on top. P.S. *No added sugar.*[48]

---

[48]Well, almost. Once again, it wouldn't be until later that we'd find out balsamic vinegar is not a vinegar in the traditional sense, but rather an aged syrup made from grapes. Fruit juice! Gak!

Sure, it looked pretty decadent, but I was petrified. What if it was awful? What if it tasted like wallpaper paste? I took a bite. Hey—wow! Happily, the girls were exclaiming as they ate—the banana ice cream was the key—perfect and sweet all on its own, creamy like the best soft-serve, and the cream and strawberries made it just the right amount more colorful and complex. I sighed a *huge* sigh of relief, and I began to think maybe, just *maybe* we'd make it through this project after all.

I know what you're wondering. Did I tell her? Did I tell Ilsa that her special birthday dessert had no *actual* added sugar in it?[49] Just to add to my fret list, I worried on this account too. I am not a fan of lying to my kids and avoid it at *almost* any cost. I can truthfully say I did *not* lie to Ilsa about her birthday dessert. Thankfully, she never asked.

February

Next up? Valentine's Day. To mark the occasion, our family's agreed-upon confection would be…chocolate mousse. Now, I had never made chocolate mousse before, but I have this unfortunate tendency to be ambitious in the kitchen at all the wrong moments. (The President is coming to dinner? Why not try grinding our own sausage for the occasion?) And because this was only our second dessert of the year, I was still in the "let's keep everyone on board!" mode—anxious to make our monthly treats fascinating enough to make everyone forget about sugar for the next four weeks. But I worried: What if it turned out deflated? Or did whatever it is that goes wrong with *mousse*? As it turned out, what was memorable

---

[49]To our knowledge.

about the chocolate mousse wasn't the night we had it, but rather the night we were *supposed* to have it.

That Valentine's Day had been a looong day. After schlepping to BJ's Wholesale to push around a shopping cart larger than a Volkswagen and read ingredients with a magnifying glass, I came back home to unload, put away, turn around, and troop back off to school and lead a two-hour afterschool activity. Finally, late that afternoon, the girls and I, all exhausted, set out to locate and purchase the only chocolate mousse ingredient my pantry lacked: heavy cream.

Dutchie's? Closed Mondays. Sheldon's? No heavy cream. Mach's Market down the road? Yes! Heavy cream hiding on the top shelf behind the half and half. Score! We hurried home so I could heat up the potato pizza leftovers from the night before and concentrate on making a beautiful Valentine's Day dessert to show my family how much I loved them and make their tummies feel all happy and full. Despite the deprivation of the "Mommy's idea" No-Sugar project, this was one of only twelve nights this year I could indulge my affection for my family in the form of a sugar-containing treat, and I was going to enjoy it, no matter how tired I was.

That was when Greta, in an effort to be helpful, read out loud the pivotal part of the recipe that I had somehow missed: "must chill for a minimum of *two hours*." What??

I stopped.

I wilted.

The dish mountain that, of late, had been growing rather ominously in the sink now loomed at me like Kilimanjaro. The potato pizza had *not* been a hit the night before and was not likely to inspire more confidence on its second trip to the dinner table. There was no bread. No time to make dessert. And everyone was *hungry*.

I wanted to lie down on the couch and cry, but it was covered with a huge pile of unfolded laundry. So instead, I stood still in the middle of the kitchen and looked lost. Fortunately for me, Steve came home at precisely that moment, recognized the look on my face, and took over. He took steaks down from the freezer for dinner, heated the potato pizza for a side dish, and handed me a pink bag with a pretty dress in it: Happy Valentine's Day. He might as well have been wearing a cape and tights.

We all felt much better after eating dinner, despite the fact that the laundry and the dishes didn't magically disappear. The kids were disappointed that our special dessert would have to wait,[50] but I explained to them that—project or no project—there is *only so much that Mommy can do*. Remind me to write that on my forehead, will you?

March

I think I may have mentioned that I'm an admitted, and only semireformed, control freak. When my friend Miles told me that she didn't just want to *make* the floral centerpieces for her own wedding, but she wanted to grow the flowers first *from seed*, *pick them*, and *then dry them* before arranging them in baskets (which I would not have put past her to have woven herself while hanging upside-down blindfolded) did *I* tell her she was crazy? No, I *completely* understood. *That's* the kind of control freak I can be.

---

[50]When we did get to enjoy it a few days hence, the chocolate mousse was fluffy and delicious and disappeared quickly. Phew.

So when the opportunity arises for me to not only make a pie from scratch, but to pick, pit, wash, and freeze the fruit myself in preparation for said pie, my first thought is not *What a lot of work!* but rather *Ooo! Where do I sign up?*

Take our family's favorite sour cherry pie. Every year in June, we know it's time to call Hick's Orchard in Granville, New York, and find out if the cherries are ready for picking. This tradition began on a Father's Day weekend many years ago when we were driving around with Steve's parents, and we stopped at the orchard on a whim. We picked a flat of the luscious red fruit, and when I got home, I found a recipe for cherry pie in my ever-reliable, broken-spined *Joy of Cooking*. We have been utterly *obsessed* with sour cherries ever since.

They're a funny thing to be obsessed with, since there's not all that much you can actually *do* with sour cherries. You can make a kick-ass pie, and you can make the Best Jam Ever, and…and…that seems to be it. That really is enough, though. In fact, every year we seem to get greedier, bringing home yet another flat piled high with the sweet-sour smelling orbs that require pitting *immediately*, because within hours of picking, they will begin to age, wrinkle, and develop icky brown-beige spots. Thus, cherry picking is an all-day event: picking is easy; pitting is hard. Well, not *hard*, but long, boring, and sticky-juice-running-down-your-forearms *annoying* when you get right down to it.

Of course, they make gadgets to make the job easier, which don't. Over the years, we've tried them all and reverted every time to the good old thumbnail technique. Remember Jack Horner sticking in his thumb and pulling out a plum? It's kind of like that—and repeat four thousand times.

In order to minimize mess, I cover the dining room table

with garbage bags and clean dishrags. Every pitter gets a station at the table and a handy supply of paper towels with which to combat Sticky Elbow Syndrome. Both of our girls are usually enthused for about the first twenty minutes, at which point they wander off and find something less mind numbing to do. Sometimes my mom is up and we'll chat while we pit; other times I've sat and pitted by myself in a Zen-like, semicomatose state until I felt encased in juice much the way I imagine a mosquito trapped in sap must feel. (Steve counts himself among the champion cherry pickers of the universe, picking one whole flat for every handful the rest of us generate, and thus rationalizes his hasty escape when I start pulling out the colanders and plastic bags. Chicken.)

Doesn't matter. I carefully wash and measure out five cups of fruit per Ziploc bag, and off they go to the deep freeze until the time comes to make a pie or perhaps a nice batch of sour-sweet jam. At any given moment, I'd guess we have about nine pies' worth of cherries in our stand-up freezer, or, as Steve would say, "Not enough!"

So I knew a cherry pie would be high on the family list of "Desert Island Desserts." After having chocolate cupcakes *and* chocolate mousse, I felt it was high time to demonstrate that dessert can exist perfectly well without chocolate, thank you.

Thus I was delighted to haul out my familiar marble rolling pin and board, drain the rich red juice from the thawed fruit, and measure out the (*gasp!*) sugar. Making the pie felt like greeting a dear friend I haven't seen in *so* long but who hasn't changed a bit. Mix defrosted fruit with sugar, add ice water to Cuisinart, roll out dough, butter the pie pan. If I have time, I always prefer to make a fancy lattice top, because it seems appropriate to the specialness of the dessert.

I usually swear under my breath later when I realize I put one of the dough strips over when it was supposed to go under, or vice versa, even though I'm certainly the only one who will ever notice.

This time, however, everything worked out just right: the lattice was perfect, I remembered to add the butter dots and brush with milk just before baking, and for once I even put on the "crust-protector" ring before the outer crust (which, being slightly higher, tends to brown much faster) was already irredeemably overdone.

Do I sound obsessed yet? Yes, I do love cherry pie. But I have to admit that it wouldn't be quite the same if we hadn't picked the fruit as a family one sunny day in June, or if I hadn't made it so many times before, always endeavoring to make it just a little more pretty, just a little more perfect—just because. There is no doubt that for me it is a labor of love.

We served the pie after dinner that night still just slightly warm and topped with a scoop of silky Wilcox vanilla ice cream. After so many weeks of No Added Sugar the blast of FRUIT with SUGAR and PASTRY—whoa! It was complete sensory overload. And it was *delicious*. The sugar went immediately to my head and made my brain feel like it was buzzing for about a half an hour. But above all, there was no question; it was *special*.

I put down my fork and felt happy, a little high, and utterly satisfied. "Now I am good," I said to no one in particular. "Now I can go another month."

I should've known, however, that something was afoot. That high feeling was my first indication that things were ever so slowly shifting: my taste buds, my body's reaction to sugar were all beginning to change.

April

By the time April came around, we were back to good old chocolate cake by request of Greta the Birthday Girl, on the occasion of her turning eleven. Fortunately, Greta wasn't having a traditional "kid" party, so all we really had to worry about was the family dessert. Phew.

The recipe I use for every chocolate-cake-requiring occasion is my grandmother's and ends up making an appearance in our house at least once a year. It's one of those funny old recipes that actually uses Crisco (gasp!) and instructs you to do all sorts of weird things like put baking soda in hot water before adding it to the batter and sour the milk by adding vinegar to it.

I love stuff like that. I love that my grandmother made this cake for my mom, my mom made this cake for me, and now I'm making it for my family. I love the weird instructions that harken back to an age when people thought nothing of taking the time to trace the cake pans with a pencil on wax paper to line the baking pans with. It's nice too, that it somehow results in a remarkably moist and not overly sweet cake that everyone seems to love. It is inevitably topped off with my mother's recipe for buttercream frosting, which is essentially a boatload of butter and powdered sugar thrown together with a teeny bit of vanilla. *That* part is awfully sweet, and every year I find myself wondering what *another* frosting might be like on my grandmother's chocolate cake (heresy!), but I haven't had the nerve to try it yet.

Of course, you only turn eleven once, so we really did it up by putting a small ball of vanilla ice cream on top of each slice. I have to admit, in addition to being delicious, the total effect was now achingly sweet to my recalibrating taste buds;

I felt instantly jittery and got a dramatic sugar rush to my head that lasted around half an hour. Oo—yuck.

Now a full four months into our Year of No Sugar, I was realizing, a firm taste shift was under way, and sweets were somehow, inexplicably, holding much, much less appeal for me. I enjoyed our monthly treat, but then also noticed that I was *paying* for it: I just felt…icky.

It wasn't till later that it occurred to me to do the math: the cake recipe called for *two* cups of granulated sugar, and the icing called for *three* cups of powdered sugar. We had divided the cake into twelve slices, so per serving that would be…holy cow! Nearly half a cup, *.41666667*, of sugar per serving!! And that's *not including the ice cream*. Well, no wonder I got a headache. It's a miracle my body didn't stage a full-scale *revolt*.

A few days later, Katrina and her kids stopped by on their way home from dinner and happened to have ice cream in the car for that night's dessert. Katrina said *of course* they would wait till they were home—they certainly wouldn't make us watch them eat ice cream while we ate that evening's No-Sugar dessert: a blueberry-and-lemon juice concoction Greta had invented while I made dinner.

Now, I was already proud of Greta's inventiveness in the pastry department, but then she *really* surprised me: "You can bring the ice cream up," she said to our friends. "*Really!* I don't mind. I had birthday cake a few days ago. I'm good!"

Well, knock me over with a feather. Things really *were* changing.

May

There were certain things I really didn't *want* to change, though. There were two favorite desserts I had no intention of going a full year without, sour cherry pie being one of them—which we had already made—and rhubarb pie being the other. Now that May was here, the funny, reddish, celery-like stalks had emerged from the ground and unfurled their giant, floppy leaves. It's a hearty, stubborn plant with a mind of its own—you accept rhubarb on its own terms or not at all. In the extended family of vegetables, rhubarb is the eccentric aunt with sunglasses and a large beach hat.

It's also one of those funny New England edibles—like gooseberries or husk cherries—that sound adorable and quaint to the uninitiated, rather like something our grand-parents might've made into a buckle or a crumble. Then, there are the devoted fans who know there are few things better than an ice-cold slice of rhubarb pie. We have two rhubarb plants in our garden—they've been here way longer than any particular homeowner—and every year we look forward to the first rhubarb pie of the season the way others look for the first robin sighting or the first blooming lilacs. It tells us that spring really has come at last.

And rhubarb and I go way back. My mom used to make rhubarb pie when I was growing up, which is weird, since we lived in the suburbs. I still have my mom's recipe, complete with her perfect five-minute Cuisinart crust, and I make it every year with an almost religious devotion. For me, eating that first bite of rhubarb sweet-sour pie is reliving a moment of childhood happiness.

So, of course, as soon as the stalks were up from the ground in spring, I set my sights on dear old rhubarb pie for our May monthly dessert. It almost came to a food fight though: Greta wanted coconut vanilla pudding cake and Ilsa had her heart set on a batch of sugar cookies. Nurturing my inner tyrant,

I decided that since neither of those choices was seasonally dependent—plus the fact that I had the distinct advantage of being the one who would actually *make* the dessert—rhubarb would prevail. Caesar lives.

———

Today we had our monthly dessert. We had rhubarb pie with Wilcox ice cream. Although I wanted coconut pudding cake, this dessert was good. The dessert days I love, but most of the time I'm not loving (the project) too much. And I'll give you three reasons.

1. Most of the time when I see something I used to like to eat, we can't have it.

2. We can't have ketchup at all—or mayonnaise. We can't have ketchup period and for mayonnaise we have aioli (which I don't particularly like).

3. At restaurants, we have to ask about everything.

—from Greta's journal

———

The funny thing about pies is how much better they can get after a day of sitting in the refrigerator, getting chilled, and letting all those sweet and sour and buttery flavors rest and meld together. Rhubarb pie is a classic example of this: out of the oven it is really, really good. Out of the fridge the next day? Ridiculous. Amazing.

And yet.

Once again, something was amiss. You'd think I'd have figured this out by now, but it was continuing to throw me every month. Finally I realized it was this…this *taste* in my mouth, like the aftertaste you get from drinking a diet soda. Bleh! What *was* that? Then I knew: It was the *sugar*. Sugar and I, it seemed, were now like old friends who hadn't seen each other in so long that when they get together it's *fun* but...a little awkward.

August

As we approached August, I realized I had a problem we hadn't encountered up to now. You see, in August, my dad's birthday falls just one day before...my mom's *boyfriend's* birthday. Ahem. (Now, I don't know much about astrology, but it seems to me that there is something going on there.)

At any rate, this year, the girls and I would be traveling to celebrate *both* of these birthdays, and fortunately for us, my mom and dad don't live too far apart for that to be possible. But if you're like me, you've already realized the unique conundrum this posed for us this year: birthday cake.

Ah, the ever-ubiquitous birthday cake. It would foil me yet.

Sooooooooo, what would be our August dessert? *Dad's* birthday cake? Or *John's* birthday cake? I pondered this. My brain resounded with the immortal wisdom of Highlander: *There can be only one!* What would we do? Uh...could we eat a half a piece of cake at each celebration? Would we skip dessert at *both* celebrations? Certainly we couldn't shun dessert at *one* birthday—that would be like choosing sides! I mean, these are two people I love in very different ways. They are apples and oranges. I'm grateful at least that their birthdays had the decency to fall one day apart, so I always have the opportunity to celebrate everyone—but this cake thing presented a new, unprecedented problem. For the first time in our entire Year of No Sugar, I had a choice to make: whose birthday got celebrated with sugar and...whose did *not*? Ack!

Ultimately, I used my understanding of the two birthday

honorees to figure it out. My dad is pretty adventurous when it comes to food and always willing to question tradition in the interest of trying something new. I knew he was interested in our family's No-Sugar project—we had had a series of conversations on the mysterious subject of what the heck we had been up to.

On the other hand, John, whose boyfriend status belies the fact that he has been with my mom for the last twenty-five years or so, is more of a person who knows what he likes and likes what he likes. For his birthday dinner, for example, we were going to the Italian restaurant that had been his favorite for the last few *decades*. He also has a very live-and-let-live philosophy—to all appearances, he is entirely neutral on the subject of our No-Sugar adventure.

Then there's my mom. Like Dad, Mom is supportive of our family project in spite of the fact that I'm pretty sure she's worried I fell on my head before coming up with the idea. Mom is the one who reads all my posts practically before I can even press "publish." Yet, she's also the one from whom I got my love of celebrations and my implicit understanding that there are just certain things you *do* to celebrate a birthday. You have a special meal. You have decorations and presents and sing the birthday song. And you have a fabulous cake.

So it was decided that Mom would order a fabulous cake from the local fabulous bakery, and that would be our "official" August dessert. Meanwhile, I was planning to make dinner for Dad at his house, so I would make him his longstanding favorite for dessert: poppy seed cake.

Without sugar.

God help me if it turned out awful. I knew Dad wouldn't mind, but *I'd* feel terrible.

But you know what? It didn't turn out awful. Dad loved it. Everybody loved it. I was astounded. No one even *asked* if there was sugar in it! Afterward, I told everyone that there was, technically speaking, no fructose/added sugar in the cake at all, and it was Dad's turn to be astounded. My seventeen-year-old brother's reaction was along the lines of "uh, yeah, whatever." *He* didn't care. Does it taste like cake? Must be cake. What I cared about was that he had eaten the whole piece—everyone had.

Now, truthfully, the cake wasn't quite as "floofy" (that's a technical term) as usual, and while we're being picky, the cream cheese frosting seemed, if anything, a bit *too* sweet to me.[51] All in all, though, I was deeply relieved and counted it a certifiable success.

And of course, the next night we had cake—*again!* Except this time it was the real-sucrose-deal. We picked up the gorgeous confection from the nearby Riviera Bakery where they are famous for fun things like Dr. Seuss–inspired shapes, edible candles, and cakes that look like giant hamburgers.[52] If you die and go to Bakery Heaven, you will likely find yourself at the Riviera—it smells like every wonderful, sweet thing you've ever eaten all at once. John's New Orleans–themed cake was a vision in purple, green, and gold, complete with

---

[51]For the modified poppy seed cake, I used dextrose in both the cake and the frosting—see the recipe section at the end of this book.

[52]As it turns out, I discovered that the mastermind behind the genius desserts at Riviera Bakehouse—and the Whimsical Bakehouse cookbooks which have sprung from it—is none other than a dear old roommate of mine from Cornell University art school—Liv Hansen. How much sense it made that Liv would combine her passion for food with her irrepressible creativity to create clever, beautiful cakes that make one feel as if you might just be consuming a masterpiece.

white chocolate Mardi Gras masks and fleur-de-lis. Inside, three thin chocolate layers were interspersed with cookies-and-cream filling. It was quite literally a work of edible art.

Perhaps predictably, it seemed overwhelmingly sweet to me. I wasn't too surprised to find that I couldn't finish my slice, and then I noticed that neither could the girls. It was *very* good, but good in the way candy is good—you only need a few bites and it's…enough.

So in the end, we were able to participate fully in both birthdays, apples *and* oranges. And we certainly got our fair share of cake. Thank goodness.

September

September was my husband's birthday month, and he had a special request. Ever since tasting it at one of Emeril's restaurants years ago, I had promised to attempt making the celebrity chef's signature dessert: banana cream pie. Steve seized this unique opportunity to bring up my long-unfulfilled commitment: I had been intimidated by the complex recipe, but how could I say no to attempting it as one of our twelve special monthly desserts? I accepted the challenge.

So Steve's birthday afternoon, I set out on my quest to conquer the banana cream pie. In Emeril's version, you first make and bake the graham cracker and mashed banana crust; then you make the pastry cream, which has to chill for two hours; after that, you place alternate layers of sliced bananas *with* pastry cream *in* the crust, then chill another two hours. Before serving, you concoct a caramel sauce of sugar, water, and heavy cream on the stove, and whip the heavy cream with vanilla and shave the chocolate, *each* of which gets ladled or dolloped or sprinkled on top just before serving.

Are you getting all of this?

In between steps, I made our actual dinner, which seemed incidental. Finally, after we had eaten dinner, opened presents, boiled the caramel, whipped the cream, and sprinkled the chocolate, we sang the birthday song, and it was time to try the pie.

Oh. My. God. Was it *SWEEEEEEEET*. It actually made my teeth hurt. I mean, go figure, right? There was only sugar in every one of those—what?—*four* separate recipes that were concocted and combined, from crust to cream filling to whipped cream to caramel drizzle. It's a wonder we didn't all pass out from Complete Sugar Shock.

Actually, I almost did. I felt *awful*. A few bites in and my head began pounding in earnest—as if it were being squeezed in a vice. The pie didn't taste right either…it was just not right at *all*. In addition to being heart-stoppingly sweet, the texture was too…*goopy*. After my entire afternoon's investment of time, I was deeply disappointed. Heartbroken. I couldn't finish my piece. Physically, I felt awful. I lay down on the couch and, exhausted, fell asleep.

It didn't help, as it turned out, that I was coming down with a cold. Still, I wondered, have I changed *so* much? I had *loved* that banana cream pie at Emeril's just as Steve had. What was happening to me? Contrary to what many had assumed, I was *not* trying to wipe desserts from the face of the earth, just making the argument that we need them to truly be special. Had I worked so hard avoiding sugar only to have my love for that occasional special dessert ruined? Is it really a case of *all* or *nothing*? I hated to admit it to myself, but lately I seemed to have become the kind of person who gets much more enjoyment out of a "dirt cookie" (as I called my bland, dextrose-sweetened, oatmeal raisin cookies, that perhaps only our family could love) than a well-made piece of pie.

Then again, I thought, isn't that what this year was all about? Changing our taste buds? Realizing that we don't "need" nearly the amount of sugar we regularly consume? Did I expect to get through the year completely unchanged? And if I did, would that be a good thing?

Oh, but change is *hard*.

The next day, despite my memory of the sickly sweetness, I tried a bite of the leftover pie. I just couldn't accept that all that work had been for nothing. But wait a minute—it was...good! Whoa—*really* good! THIS actually reminded me of the pie we had had all those years ago at Emeril's. After the extra hours in the fridge, the correct texture had finally been reached, and the coldness had additionally softened the sweety sweetness. I was relieved: perhaps I *hadn't* lost my ability to enjoy a good sweet after all.

Later that night after dinner, I shared the last pie slice with my husband. I should've stuck with the one or two bites though. After that, it started seeming overly sweet again. Afterward, I had to go gargle just to get that overpowering taste out of my mouth. And, alas, the headache came back.

I wondered if the legacy of this No-Sugar Year for me would be a two-bite limit on all desserts. Although my body would surely thank me for it, I had to admit, I was more than a little ambivalent about that.

November

Ah, Thanksgiving. The mother of all quintessentially American holidays and—not coincidentally—the mother of all gluttonous holidays as well.

It's kind of amazing all the different foods that we're supposed to concoct in order to have a "real" or "traditional" Thanksgiving. It's daunting. In fact, I have a dear friend whose family bags the whole thing and makes a large Thanksgiving pizza.

As we all know, the beleaguered turkey-day host isn't responsible for *just* turkey and stuffing and mashed potatoes—oh no!—but cranberries, gravy, and whatever other sides you grew up eating *with* them: maybe peas, corn, applesauce; maybe green bean casserole with the crunchy canned onions on top or strawberry Jell-O with little banana UFOs floating inside, or perhaps yam casserole drenched in brown sugar, butter, and tiny marshmallows…No matter what, everyone seems to have a food it Just Wouldn't Be Thanksgiving Without. (Guilty! For me it is my mom's oyster stuffing. It. Is. So. Good.)

So once you get through making all the mandatory foods, the "it wouldn't be Thanksgiving without" foods, and anything special or new that you decided to throw in this year, you've got yerself a fairly serious Mount Everest of *food*.

However, despite the fact that it was a ridiculous starch fest (more stuffing with your mashed potatoes, my dear?) and the fact that many of those "traditional" dishes can practically cause instant diabetes (Mini marshmallows? Did the pilgrims have those?), despite *all that*, our family hosted (read: not just us palate-altered folks, but *normal* people too!) and got through the entire meal No-Sugar style.[53] Yes! Really! Well, how the heck did we do that?

---

[53] That is, soup to nuts, but not dessert—Thanksgiving dessert would be our November sugar-containing dessert.

First of all, gravy is always a prime suspect for hiding sugar—but my mom bought it at Whole Foods and checked the ingredients, so we were safe on that account. She also made that green bean casserole with the crunchy onions on top, and I was amazed to find only dextrose(!), not sugar or any icky variant thereof, in the ingredient list. Well, yay! Not that this was health food you understand, but still.

My proudest achievement of the day, however, was my no-added-sugar cranberry sauce, which I had practiced earlier in the week just to be *sure* they would meet everyone's Official Turkey Day Fruit expectations. I mean, these might be the only cranberries some of our guests would eat all year! In the making, I was amazed on many counts:

1. Making cranberry sauce was *ridiculously* easy. Because everyone I know always buys those cans of jellied stuff saturated with high-fructose corn syrup, I'd gotten the impression it must be rocket science. Instead, it's about as easy as making oatmeal.

2. I was *very* stressed about gaining the correct amount of sweetness and jellylike texture. The problem was solved by cooking the berries in a mixture of boiling water and dextrose, and then adding a healthy dollop of one of my newest favorite things: glucose syrup. More on that in a minute.

3. Did you know cranberries *pop* when you cook them? How much fun is that?

So, right around this time, I had gone in search of another non-fructose sweetener: *glucose syrup*. David Gillespie had used it in one of the recipes on his website that I wanted to make. I know what you're thinking. *Glucose syrup?* It sounded scary, like an ingredient for a science experiment involving frogs and tweezers. And it sounded even *less* appetizing than dextrose, if that was possible. Hmm. But I *really* wanted to make the granola bar recipe, and my previous attempt to do without had resulted in granola bar confetti. It was delicious, but it just didn't hold together at all.

So, as with dextrose powder, I found it online. I purchased a tiny tub of the mysterious stuff, which arrived looking more like something for my car engine than food. Glucose syrup is clear, gooey, and tarlike in consistency, and it gets absolutely *everywhere* when you try to measure it. *Yuck*—I thought—*this is not the kind of ingredient anyone was going to want to lick the spoon of.* Then again, I reasoned, Gillespie had never steered us wrong yet.

And of course, he was right: glucose syrup is the perfect solution for anything that needs not only sweetening, but also the viscous thickening that many traditional sweeteners provide, like molasses or honey, for example. More and more lately, I'd been using dextrose powder, to the point where I would actually almost forget that I was making any modification. If the recipe called for half a cup of sugar, I read "three-quarter cup dextrose." But there are situations where dextrose alone just isn't going to create that thick texture you need. Enter: glucose syrup. Wearing a white hat. The cranberries are *saved*!

Most significantly, our sugar dessert for the month was to be our Thanksgiving pumpkin pie. But because, as I described, I had gotten so *used* to my big orange container, I completely forgot at first and used dextrose in the crust rather than actual sugar. When I got around to mixing the pumpkin with the spices, I had to remind myself—*go get the* **actual** *sugar, Eve.*

The pie was delicious, as pumpkin pie always is. It only takes three-quarters of a cup of sugar in the entire recipe, so compared to many desserts, the sweetness is fairly mild and not likely to cause us all banana-cream-pie-style headaches. Actually, our monthly dessert passed with such little fanfare that it made me wonder—have we entered a new stage here, where sugar just didn't *matter* so much anymore? Could it be, after eleven months of diligence, and with the help of magical ingredients such as dextrose and glucose syrup, that we had gotten to a place where we were conditioned to be perfectly happy with a vastly reduced level of sweet? Had we really, at last, shunned sugar?

And I couldn't help but also wonder: if I *had* used dextrose in the pie filling too, would anyone have noticed?

CHAPTER 13

HALLOWEEN
WITHOUT CANDY

C rap!" I banged the steering wheel with my palm. "Rats!"
It was mid-October and I was driving back to
Vermont after meeting with one of the sources of great
inspiration for this project: David Gillespie.

Everything had gone great. I mean, how lucky was I?
I'd been corresponding with Gillespie via email ever since
he happened to notice I was blogging and tweeting endless effusive compliments about his book *Sweet Poison.*[54]
Holy crap! I had thought—David Gillespie read *my* review
of his book? This was like…like serving cupcakes to
Martha Stewart!

So I managed to rearrange my schedule (and that of my
family) soon after I found out he was going to be in New
York City for a few days and had offered to meet up with
me. The chance to meet the man who wrote, "If obesity was
a disease like bird flu, we'd be bunkered down with a shotgun

---

[54]And I'm not done, either: It's *still* the very best book out there by far for those
who want a thorough layperson's explanation of what it is exactly that sugar
does in your body and why. Also, he's hilarious.

and three years' supply of baked beans in the garage"? I mean, how could I pass *that* up?

Of course, getting to *anywhere* from Vermont is a bit of a task, but since I wasn't planning on being in *his* stomping grounds (Australia) anytime very soon, it seemed like a unique opportunity. So, dressed up and bleary-eyed, I left home at 6:45 a.m., drove to the suburb of White Plains, hopped on the 11:05 commuter train, and was dumped out in Grand Central in time to meet him for lunch at one p.m. Phew!

In fact, I was early. *Really* early. And nervous. I started to have *what if* thoughts. What if…he thinks I'm a *moron*? What if this lunch will necessitate an involved conversation about GLUT proteins and the role of the hypothalamus? What if my writing is waaaay more interesting than I am in person?

I know, I know. But these are the things one worries about when you get to the restaurant where you're supposed to be meeting one of your big inspirations and you have a full *hour* to get anxious. I was just deeply grateful that my car hadn't failed me, the train hadn't been late, I hadn't gotten lost, I didn't feel nauseous, and it wasn't a bad hair day.

And of course, I needn't have worried. David Gillespie, I am happy to report, is about as easygoing a guy as you're going to encounter. He's reserved, witty, and quietly passionate about his work. Like me, he's the kind of person who prefers to state his case in print and let others make of it what they will, and who isn't especially fond of having to sell people on his ideas in person.

In fact, he didn't start out to make a No-Sugar movement at all. Rather, he said, when folks were curious how he had managed to lose such a tremendous amount of weight, he would reply, "I stopped eating sugar."

"Well, of course, *that* wasn't good enough!" Gillespie laughed over lunch. "So I decided to write *Sweet Poison*. And then I could tell them to read *that*!"

And the book's power to convince has worked well. It worked *so* well that Gillespie has sold over a hundred thousand copies of *Sweet Poison* in Australia and many more of the follow-up companion book *The Sweet Poison Quit Plan*. In fact, the motivation for this very trip was to find a publisher to distribute these same volumes in the U.S.[55]

I was amazed to hear David's stories. For example, in Gillespie's children's school, in addition to making provisions for children with allergies and food sensitivities, they now make provisions for kids who aren't eating sugar. Let me say that again: *They make provisions for the children who aren't eating sugar.* As many as ten different children in a single grade level.

!!!!

By way of contrast, I related the story of Greta's recent standardized testing at school, which went on for three days, the by-product of which was a tiny *mountain* of treat wrappers that she dutifully carried home for me to see. "And this doesn't include the ice cream every day!" she added helpfully.

It's been so tempting. I've just given up trying to stay away from it at school.

—from Greta's journal

---

[55]Turns out, my copy had been purchased from a reseller on Amazon. If you are looking for it, be careful not to confuse Gillespie's *Sweet Poison* (published by Penguin in Australia) with the American book of the same title by Dr. Janet Hull, which is on the dangers of aspartame.

Shortly after this event—just to carry this tangent one step farther—our family was paying a visit to the local farmer's market and there was candy bloody *everywhere* in anticipation of the upcoming Halloween festivities. At this point, despite telling myself everyone's intentions were kind, I was starting to get a little peeved. "What, do they not think they'll be getting enough candy *tomorrow*?" I muttered. "Is an entire *pillowcase full* not enough??" After repeatedly demurring the bowl of cheap treats that was proffered at nearly every single table, one fellow held out a bowl of brightly colored hot peppers to us, causing us to do a double take. He laughed and apologized for not having candy. He assured us that the *next* table had candy.

"Yes," I said grimly. "There's *always* candy!"

Lucky for Gillespie (who is father to six children, all of whom are subsisting undeprived on No Sugar) they don't *have* Halloween in Australia. They also don't have high-fructose corn syrup. But they *do* have all the same sugar-related health problems as Americans (diabetes, heart disease, obesity, etc.), which surely negates the argument that HFCS is any worse than plain old familiar sugar.

I learned this, and so many other interesting things, at our lunch. I learned that balsamic vinegar *isn't* really vinegar and *is* fortified with sugar. I learned that Crisco was invented in 1911. I learned that Gillespie's next two books would detail what he feels is the other great dietary scourge of our time: seed oils. (Canola, vegetable, corn, hydrogenated oils, etc.[56])

---

[56]Those books are now out and titled *Big Fat Lies* and *Toxic Oil*, both published by Penguin Australia.

According to Gillespie, these are even harder to ferret out than sugar and are the other missing piece of our health puzzle, namely cancer. Whoa.

I learned that Gillespie and I had read all the same books and that his first book was tentatively titled *Raisin Hell* because somebody somewhere got confused and thought the book was about the dangers of "fruit toast." (Get it? Fructose? Ha ha!!)

And I thoroughly enjoyed having lunch with perhaps one of the only people on the planet who would nod knowingly when I blurt out, "And what's the deal with *agave*!?!"

So why *was* I so annoyed on the drive home? I realized, way belatedly, that I had completely forgotten the bloggers code: Always. Take. Pictures. Did I take a picture of me and him? Did I take a picture of what we ate? The restaurant? The bum outside? *Anything???* Nope. You know, sometimes it's a wonder I manage to leave the house with my head still attached. Oh well.

SO, where *do* two No-Sugar proponents eat for lunch in New York City? We ate at Les Halles (fittingly, the restaurant of another of my favorite writers, Anthony Bourdain). We had some very nice steaks and French fries, and a side salad... with no dressing.

––––––––

As it turns out, David Gillespie wasn't the only interesting person I got to meet as a consequence of the No-Sugar Project. Back in March while flying with my dad en route to Mayo clinic, I happened to look up from my seat in the first row of coach to see someone I recognized sitting in first class. I did a double take, the way you do to be sure you aren't seeing things, and then I knew. *Holy cow! That's* mother freaking Jason Jones!

For those of you who are not rabid fans of the political humor show *The Daily Show*, Jason Jones is one of the primary correspondents who regularly delivers news stories "on location"—in front of a green screen in Comedy Central's New York City studio. My husband and I are big, huge, ENORMOUS fans of the show, so of course, I texted Steve right away to tell him. It's Jason Jones! It's Jason Jones! The one who's married to Samantha Bee! (also a Daily Show correspondent) Sitting not five seats away from me! Holy crap!! What do I do?!

I had meant it rhetorically, of course. There was nothing to *do*. I'm not the autograph-seeking type, so of course I sat there and admired my mere proximity to a fairly famous person, period. And then suddenly, I *knew*. My heart sank and started beating fast simultaneously. There was something I should do. Aw, *man...*

I had to tell him about the No-Sugar Project.

Shit.

But I *knew* I had to do it—I knew it with as much conviction as I had known, way back on that day I had watched Dr. Lustig's YouTube lecture, that we had to try living without sugar for a year. It's almost as if the idea had come from outside of me, rather than from me: *This was what had to happen.* We had to eat for a year without sugar—we had to try. And I had to write about it. I was possessed, obsessed, and this was the only cure.

It was in this way that I *knew* I had to talk to Jason Jones. Why? Because what if they just *happened* to be doing a story next week on one of the controversial proposed soda taxes?

Or a story on projected obesity rates in America? Or a story on Michelle Obama's recent and much-touted "Let's Move" healthy kids initiative? I mean, this story, the story of the fattening of America, was all over the news with increasing frequency. Wouldn't I be remiss not to try to get the No-Sugar message out there?

No, I'd never forgive myself if I didn't try. In fact, I'd forever blame everything that ever happened in the rest of my life on this one, quintessential failure of fortitude: My No-Sugar blog dwindled sadly into obscurity? Should've introduced myself to Jason Jones. I broke down and ate an entire sugar sculpture minutes before midnight on New Year's Eve? Too bad I hadn't talked to Jason Jones. My watch stopped? Jason Jones could've fixed it.

I took deep breaths. Have I mentioned I'm no good in person? There's a reason I'm a writer you know. I thought about what I needed to say. I didn't even have a business card with me—curses!—so I ripped a sad little piece of paper out of my notebook and scrawled my name and blog address on it. I took more deep breaths.

After the plane was well in the air and beverage service had been through, I stood up and walked the few steps to first class. I walked right past Jason Jones. I went to the lavatory.

On the way back, though, I knew it was my last chance. I couldn't keep going to the lavatory and eyeing Jason Jones like a stalker. I had to say something. I tried not to think, because if I thought, I wouldn't have done it.

"Hello," I said. "Are you, by any chance, Jason Jones?"

Well, of course he was.

I introduced myself. I told him what a big fan I was—of him and of his wife. I told him my husband was going to be terribly jealous that I had met him. And then I paused. I got really quiet. I did my best to sound like a totally sane person who is definitely not a serial killer. And I told him I had a project I was working on which might be of interest.

Moments later, I was talking with both Jones and a fellow across the aisle whose name I should've caught—I really should get an *award* for how bad I am at this—who produces all the sketches Jason is in.

"He's really the brains behind everything," Jason said. (The two of us being on a first-name basis and all, you know.) He added self-deprecatingly, "I'm just the monkey in the suit."

They wanted to know the same things everybody else wanted to know, but I could tell they were prodding for any comic potential.

"Have you lost any weight?"

"What does your husband say?"

"How do the kids feel about it? Are they any calmer? Have they freaked out?"

I tried to give them hilarious, fascinating answers, but— and stop me if I've already mentioned this—I'm not so especially fascinating or hilarious in person. Plus, at this point, we were a mere eight weeks in to the Year of No Sugar—we'd barely dipped our toes in the water.

But I tried. I had an actual, real conversation in which polite laughter occurred, and they took my pathetic little piece of paper. They were awfully nice, considering that they probably get accosted fourteen times a day by people who want to tell them about how their family is living on a trapeze to protest circus apathy or something.

I went back to my seat and I felt great. I had done it—I had *tried*, despite being intimidated down to the last fiber of my being. Nothing ever did come of it—well, not *yet*! Can you hear me, JASON??—but I had done my best, despite myself. No Sugar was teaching me things about myself I never could've imagined.

All I can say is it's a good thing Michelle Obama wasn't on my plane, or I probably would've had to request oxygen.

But back to Halloween.

Halloween was going to be a big milestone in our Year of No Sugar. I knew this because it was one of the very first questions asked when we introduced the idea of our family project in the car ride home from Grandma's house lo those many months ago.

"But what about *Halloween*? What about *Christmas*?" my children had wailed from the backseat. I was ruing the day I ever came up with this plan already, and we hadn't even started.

"We'll figure it out," I had said in what I hoped was my most-convincing mom voice. "Don't worry. We'll do it together. As a family. And it's not forever."

My kids were thoroughly un-reassured as we snuffled our red-eyed way home. I realized then that I was going to have to give momentous annual sugar festivities, such as Halloween, some very serious thought.

So in the days approaching the end of October, I began canvasing every parent I knew about creative Halloween strategies. I came across several methods for dealing with the autumnal sugar onslaught, this mother-of-all-candy holidays. Let me count the ways…

• The ol' switcheroo: my friend Miles said that in Dayton,

Ohio, the "Switch Witch" comes to visit many houses the night after Halloween, leaving toys in place of sweets.

- The "out of sight, out of mind" policy: I'm pretty sure my own mom ascribed to this one, in which we would eat one piece of candy after dinner for a week or so, and then we'd forget all about it. The remainder would, I'm quite certain, end up in the trash well before it was time to worry about pumpkin pie and cranberry sauce.

- There's always bribery. On NPR, I heard a story about a dentist who was offering to *buy* the candy to keep it out of kids' mouths. The going rate was a dollar per pound, up to five pounds. Not bad.

- I found one local family who opts out altogether. They stay home and pick a special family dessert to make instead.

Even if you're not convinced that sugar is a toxin, most parents do seem to get that consuming candy on Halloween-scale is not good. Maybe it's because of the unfortunate kid every year at the parade or the party who overdoes it and throws up, or maybe we just know, instinctively, that consuming a pillowcase full of *anything*, anything at *all*, can't be good.

Here's what we always used to do when I was a kid: after trick-or-treating till our lips turned blue from the late October air ("*But Mo-oooom!* If I wear my coat no one can see my *costume!!*"), we'd all congregate on the floor of someone's living room and pour our bags of cheap treats out to sort and count and trade. I always liked this part the best—we were like little pirates, or maybe bankers, gleefully portioning out the gold coins.

And now that I have kids, they do this too. On Halloween night of our Year of No Sugar, we *did* go trick-or-treating as always, with a gaggle of kids racing ahead and the dutiful parents lagging behind. At the end, we all trooped back to Katrina's house where the kids immediately took over the living room by dumping several tons of high-fructose corn syrup in a variety of colorful wrappers onto the carpet. A frenzy of sorting and showing off and bartering began.

"I have NERDS!"

"Look! A *mint-flavored* Milky Way!"

"What are *these?*"

"*Who* gives out *barbecue chips?*"

"Oo! What do you want for your *Sour Patch Kids?*"

Meanwhile, Katrina's dog, Inky, was wasting no time. Ignoring the candy completely, he made like a Hoover vacuum when an entire baggie filled with popcorn ended up on the floor, deftly maneuvering around the Tootsie Rolls and tiny boxes of Junior Mints.[57]

I laughed when I saw that our friend Robin had brought homemade cupcakes along for everyone. It reminded me of the farmer's market the previous Saturday, where the vendors were plying my children with candy, pressing Starbursts and hard candies into our hands before we could say no.[58]

Despite this prophetic handwriting on the wall, I had been nonetheless astounded earlier that Halloween day to walk into Greta's sixth-grade classroom and find all the kids having a Halloween treat consisting of a sugar doughnut and

---

[57]So what happened to all that candy once we got home to *our* house? The kids each got to pick one candy to have that night with their friends, and the rest went to the very, very back of the tip-toppest shelf in our kitchen food cupboard. It is still there.

[58]Sometimes it's just easier to smile and say thank you. They went directly into the trash when we got home.

a large handful of assorted candy. My eyes got big. What? Did they not feel tonight was going to be sufficient? Did they have to be *primed* with sugar pre-event too?

If I had never noticed it before, I certainly noticed it now: people just can't seem to help themselves when it comes to the idea of making a child happy. And what easier way to make a child happy than with an inexpensive little bit of sugar? Of course, the problem is, it's *too* easy, so everyone, *everyone*, EVERYONE gets into the act. Robin's adorable homemade cupcakes aren't really the problem; it's all the junk that likely came before that—and will likely come after that too.

My sugar-distant vantage point was giving me a unique view of the holiday season, and I was shocked at what I saw. I realized that it had become *so* cheap and *so* easy to hand a child a treat that inflation had set in. No longer is it sufficient for the teacher to bring the kids each a doughnut—there has to be a pile of candy next to it. No longer is it sufficient for kids to get a single treat at each house; now many houses go to the trouble of packing little paper candy bags full of *several treats each*. No longer is it sufficient to have a treat or two (or fourteen) from the candy bag that night; we have to provide *dessert* on top of that. Because what else do you do? It's Halloween! Or Christmas! Or Valentine's Day! Or somebody's birthday! Or you're just feeling depressed! Or happy! You see what I'm getting at here.

When we met, *Sweet Poison* author David Gillespie told me that he's always interested to watch what happens to American kids after Halloween: they all start getting sick. Sure, you could blame it on the change of temperature, more time spent inside in closer quarters, yadda yadda, but what if it's *not* just those things? Would we all be so quick to dole out those easy-to-come-by bits of happiness to children if we knew it was going to hinder their immune systems? Would we view it the way we view the WWII practice of handing out free cartons of cigarettes to soldiers now?

Then again, I can't help it; I still love Halloween. Every year, I spend much of the month of October getting ready for it, picking out costume patterns and fabric with my children, and then sewing like a madwoman. When the appointed night comes, we venture forth, armed with flashlights and reflective tote bags and cameras, not to mention the optional umbrellas or long underwear. We tromp around the village with our friends, often running into other friends and joining up like packs of amiable, gaudily dressed, and highly super-vised wild animals.

Then this year, of all years, the most amazing thing hap-pened. Early on, our group had effectively snowballed to an impressive size—perhaps thirty or more adults and kids found ourselves congregated in the parking lot of the fire department. And out of nowhere *something* was happening. Grown-ups were yelling, "Stop! Stop! Everybody come over here! Everybody join hands!"

As we all looked around blankly, trying to discern what exactly was going on, it became clear that my friend Sue was orchestrating something. All thirty or so of us, large and small, costumed and not, put down our flashlights and bags of candy and obediently joined hands.

Once we were all in an enormous circle, Sue had us let go hands at just one spot, so we formed a curved line. Then she began walking around the interior of our circle, making a spiral inward, inward. And because we had all joined hands, we were all walking too, following her, passing each other, giggling and making faces and talking to one another animatedly.

Once she got to the middle-middle-middle and could go no further she turned one hundred eighty degrees and began to walk a spiral back out again. Have you ever done this game? It seems like something I must've done at camp or elementary school or something, but never, never had I done it on a moonlit night in the parking lot of the fire department with a group of parents and children I love so well. And never before with a group of tiny Mad Hatters and queens and monkeys and fairies and zombie monsters. As we spun around and around the wheel of our friends and children, it felt like we had joined the witches themselves to perform a rite of autumn. It felt positively pre-Christian.

Isn't it something like this—that is so much harder to achieve than that fleeting bit of happiness that comes in a plastic wrapper—that we really *want* from our holidays? A sense of connection, of community, of ritual, of transformation? I'm sympathetic with my friends who opt out, celebrating at home on Halloween. I understand it. But I really don't *want* to stay home, on Halloween or any other holiday for that matter, because that feels to me like hiding. I want to be able to go out and celebrate with my friends, with my kids' friends, with my community. Unfortunately, our culture doesn't seem to remember much about how you celebrate things without buying a bunch of unnecessary stuff and without consuming a bunch of unnecessary sugar.

I thought Sue's pagan circle was a brilliant way to remind us.

CHAPTER 14

FOOD TIME TRAVEL

By November, I was starting to get the feeling that we were going back in time, cleaning our cast-iron pan, gathering the eggs from our chickens, buying our milk from the local farm in half-gallon mason jars, selecting apples out of wooden bins at the farmer's market, ordering bread from our local general store. Our freezer was full of meat: half a cow and half a pig locally raised and slaughtered. At a restaurant supply house, I was buying butter by the thirty-six-pound case and flour by the fifty-pound bag. One day, I realized I really needed something from the actual supermarket and I felt kind of...disappointed.

It wasn't entirely intentional; it just seemed to be the natural evolution of things when one tries to get away from processed foods (read: added-sugar foods). Want good bread? If you aren't prepared to make it in the quantity your family will consume, you order it from Jed in Rupert, who makes the area's best no-sugar bread with only four ingredients. Want organic meat? Unless you want to remortgage your house to buy it at the farmer's market, or pick over the sad, nonexistent selection at our local supermarkets (no Whole Foods out here!), you find a guy who knows a cow and a reputable slaughterhouse. And so on.

As if to complete the effect, for a birthday present, my husband had arranged something I've *always* wanted to do: a hearth-cooking workshop. So early one Saturday morning I, and six friends, converged on the historic homestead of Sally Brillon in Hebron, New York.

As we walked up the path in the crisp morning air, I looked around at the ancient outbuildings—remnants of the many different jobs having a family farm used to entail. Standing on the flagstone step, we knocked on the saltbox door and entered another world.

I was in heaven. Immediately upon entering, we were warmed by waves emanating from the enormous slate hearth that dominated the room. Sally had started the fire two hours earlier, to get it up to the temperatures we'd be needing to cook our meal for the day: roast chicken, potatoes with parsley, mashed Hubbard squash, cranberries, bread, and apple pie for dessert. We seven students and Sally spent the next five hours accomplishing this task.

I will admit, I am a little obsessed with this time period. If PBS ever does *Frontier House* again, I will politely beat people out of the way with a large stick to volunteer.[59] Why do I love this stuff so much? I wonder. After all, we are talking about the age when the average lifespan for a woman was, like, twelve or something. And of course, we must remember Sally was making the experience all quite painless for us; *we* didn't have to stoke the fire at 7 a.m. *We* didn't have to wash

---

[59]Did you ever see this show? In 2002, three families had to establish homesteads and live as if it were the year 1883. Now that's *my* kind of reality television.

the cast-iron pans and dishes for eight afterward in a tub of lukewarm water. She had a *real* bathroom for us, and none of us were in danger of dying from appendicitis, childbirth, or from an infected scab on the knee. We had it sooooo easy.

Instead, we got to do the fun part: we cooked two chickens in a reflecting oven before the fire, turning the spit every fifteen minutes. We boiled pots full of vegetables that hung from S hooks off a crane that swung into place over the flames. We started a soft wood fire in the bake oven and filled it with red coals until it was ready to bake our two loaves of bread. Lastly, after assembling a lovely apple pie, we laid it carefully in a cast-iron pot, placed it on a "burner" of hot coals directly on the hearth, and then shoveled coals on the lid—after a time, those coals would be removed and replaced with fresh. It was *really* starting to smell good in there.

And as you can imagine, when it was all done and we were seated around a table set with china and candles, it *tasted* good too. Not gourmet, not fancy-recipe good, but *good*. Wholesome. Filling. Real.

I loved that we used pot lid lifters and tin ladles and yellowware bowls. There was no Teflon, no plastic, no mixers or microwaves. In fact, there was only *one* modern toxin that I could see: sugar.

Of course, you must've already guessed there was sugar in the cranberries and in the apple pie. For good measure, Sally's recipe also had us drizzle maple syrup onto the top of the mashed squash. After some thought, I had decided ahead of time not to request any recipe changes—it was authenticity we were going for here, after all. The cranberries tasted almost painfully sweet to me, but the squash and the pie were very mildly sweet, even to my recently more sensitive tongue. Sally later told me that one class she had actually left the sugar out of the pie by mistake and nobody even noticed—it was just as good.

Back in those days, sugar was a lot harder to come by and boiling your own maple syrup was a task that took up a considerable portion of one's spring energies. As we waited for the chicken and bread loaves to finish baking, Sally read to us snippets from the diaries of John Quincy Wilson, who lived in that very house in the late 1800s with his wife and three children. A few entries described the gargantuan undertaking of making maple syrup: sterilizing the sap buckets, soaking the wood barrels in the nearby stream to expand the wood to seal any cracks, gathering the sap bucket by bucket, and finally building the arch for the long evaporating process, not in a sap house like today, but actually out in the open air of the woods. If only sugar was that hard to come by nowadays.

So, I got to live out my Laura Ingalls fantasy, at least for a morning. Too bad my 1840s-era house isn't *quite* old enough to have had a cooking hearth of its own. Sally tells me that during that time period, they likely used a cast-iron stove. (Hmmmmm—I wonder what *that* would be like?)[60]

All in all, it's safe to say I have a moderate-to-severe case of food curiosity. Not the kind that would secure me a spot eating pigeon feet or yak eyeballs on the Food Network or anything, mind you, but still.

This wasn't always the case, however, which brings me to the story of the time I didn't eat goat.

It was just before my husband and I were married and my mother had given us the incredible engagement gift of

---

[60]You can see how I get into trouble.

a week's safari in Tanzania. I know, right? Steve and I and nine other travelers bumping along dirt "roads" and taking four million snapshots of elephants and zebras. It was unlike anything I had ever done before—or have done since.

I felt *incredibly* young, which at the age of twenty-six I certainly was, especially compared to all the other participants on the trip. To make matters more interesting, I was the only person on the trip who, at that time, didn't eat red meat or poultry.

Our camps were primitive enough that we slept in tents and our bread was baked in a pot buried in the ground. Nonetheless, our tour leader, Justin, somehow made sure that I—the lone pescatarian—had a lovely little plate of fish and vegetables to eat every night at dinner. Then one night, several of our tour companions were feeling bored and restless. They felt we weren't getting an "authentic" enough experience and requested a meal that would've been eaten by the locals: goat.

Consequently, a day or two later, a live goat (shall we call him Fred?) was purchased and tied up near the dining tent where we listened to it lowing and bleating throughout lunch. To my sensitive, vegetarian ears, it sounded as if a doomed soul was mourning its impending fate—although in retrospect I imagine it was just as possible that it simply didn't care to be tied up in the hot sun.

Later I was told that the goat was killed in traditional fashion, using a blood bowl into which the goat's slit neck emptied, after which it was roasted and served in a traditional saucy stew. Fred Stew.

I was trying very hard not to think about that anthropomorphized goat I had conjured up in my head who, I was sure, had hopes and dreams and a family of twelve to support at home. I was irked at my traveling companions for initiating such a violent endeavor for the simple purpose of their amusement, and even more annoyed when they were unimpressed with the novelty of the meal. To me they seemed like spoiled Roman noblemen who were miffed that the gladiators hadn't died in an interesting enough manner.

That was fifteen years ago. It's amazing how much a person can change in that time. Given the same scenario again today, I would surely be the first in line to watch the ritual goat slaughter. I would be excited to try the cassoulet du goat, and who knows? Perhaps I would even be persuaded to try a sip from the blood bowl—the Massai ritualistically mix the blood with milk and drink it, you know.

At any rate, I would be fascinated, and it surely would be the high point of a pretty amazing trip, rather than a low point. (I left lunch early that day, feeling queasy after listening to the crying goat and the laughing Roman noblemen for twenty minutes.)

So why the drastic change? Have I lost my compassion? Do I no longer feel empathetic for animals? No, I still have a deep and abiding respect for animals and believe that they have real emotions and feel real pain. What changed for me is twofold: first, as I mentioned in an earlier chapter, I realized how much healthier and stronger I felt when I was consuming meat—a hard fact to argue with.

Second, I read an interview with a philosopher who talked about the nature of life—the very process of being—as inherently destructive on some level. The only way to ensure that our existence creates *no* harm in the world is…not to exist. *Whoa.* There was more to it than that, but that was the gist: I kill stuff (whether actively or passively), therefore I am. For the first time in twenty years of meat avoidance, I wondered: Is abstaining from meat more hypocritical than helpful? Was I pretending to help the world while denying the fact that my very existence caused, by extension, the death of animals, plants, insects, and microorganisms all the time?

Another of my favorite writers, the farmer-philosopher Joel Salatin agrees: "The most inhumane perspective is the one that denies the life-death-decay-regeneration cycle. Everything is constantly eating and being eaten."[61]

I decided that I had no plans to benefit the universe by jumping off the nearest cliff, thank you. The alternative was to come to the realization that nature had it right: living, and in particular *eating*, involves some degree of violence by definition. We can deny that fact and limp along, sucking on wheatgrass and feeling lousy, or we can embrace it and handle our animals in a manner that is healthy, kind, and respectful.

Currently I feel that the greatest act of respect we can have for animals is to let them *be* animals—whether wild or domesticated—for whatever the duration of their life may be. As a born-again carnivore, what that means to me is trying to eat only meat that had a pretty happy life, which means no feed lots, no living in a cage in the dark, no animals hopped up on pharmaceutical cocktails. Unfortunately, this is not very easy and often not terribly cheap either. But I think it's the right approach, the ethical approach, and, not coincidentally, the approach closest to what our ancestors have done historically.

There it is again—that idea of food history, which seemed to keep cropping up. If the problem of sugar had increased as a result of the pursuit of "progress" (industrial production,

---

[61]Joel Salatin, Correspondance, *The Sun*, January, 2013.

convenience foods), then could it be that the sugar antidote was to be found in looking backward? What, I wondered, would that look like? Probably a lot like the traditional family farm.

Although the idea of the self-sufficient family farm is something of an anachronism these days, I have some friends who attempt it with the help of the modern-day convenience of a chest freezer.

Randy and Annie are the friends I mentioned earlier who, amazingly and single-handedly, raise and slaughter fifty-two organic chickens for their family's consumption every year.

As it happened, one summer day, Annie mentioned that they were going to be "processing" (the appropriate euphemism) their birds the following weekend. So I asked what, for me, was the next logical question: "Can I come?"

Annie left the decision up to Randy, who is the one who does the majority of the processing on the appointed day. A few days later, I caught up with Randy, but at first he seemed a little tentative.

"If you don't mind my asking," he said, "*why* do you want to do this?" Funny, my husband asked me much the same question, and with a very odd look on his face too, come to think of it. Was it *that* bizarre a request? I wondered. It wasn't as if I had proposed we take a school field trip to the local funeral parlor or anything. (My husband actually did that as a child. Fun! Is this where they keep the embalming fluid, mister?) I mean, honestly, how bad could it really be? Was there something I was missing here? I wondered if I should reconsider my request.

Would slimy chicken parts be flying everywhere? Blood spurting, cartoon fashion in every direction? Would I beat a hasty retreat back to vegetarianism, ruined forever after for any appreciation of fine poultry? Would I sob uncontrollably/ be scarred for life/suffer terrible, flailing-chicken nightmares? Would I (and this was important) lose my lunch?

It is definitely interesting to see the spectrum of reactions one gets in this day and age—even in Vermont—to the idea of voluntarily killing a defenseless animal. Hunting, of course, is a similar topic, and the few hunters we know are noticeably shy on the details, feeling out whether the person they are speaking to will respond to a hunting story with sincere enthusiasm or wide-eyed horror.

Perhaps then, raising birds for meat and dispatching them methodically holds even more potential revulsion. I mean, at least the deer had a fighting chance, right? After generations of being bred to be docile, sedentary, and fat, the meat bird is...How shall I say this politely? None too bright. There ain't no fight-or-flight going on here, people. Mostly it's just sit-and-stare.

So, Randy agreed to call me when he was down to the last batch of chickens late Sunday. That afternoon, I cleaned the kitchen and waited for the phone to ring. It was a weird feeling, this aimless waiting, as if a baby was about to be born when, in fact, it was really quite the opposite situation.

Then again, I thought, something *is* being born today: food. Real food—not that ersatz stuff they try to pass off as food at the gas station or even the supermarket, but the real McCoy, the way our ancestors knew it for generations. Food that is the result of your own work, by your own hands, that doesn't attempt to deny or obscure the essence of what it is: a dead animal.

It makes sense that the more honest we are about this, the better. The factory farm industry is more than happy to take advantage of our modern squeamishness and our collective cultural agreement to suspend our disbelief. (We all *know* it is a dead animal—buuuut let's pretend it's not!) If you haven't been to one, let's just say there's a really good reason they don't have school field trips to industrial chicken farms. (Pretty much the same reason they don't have school field trips to funeral parlors: too many nightmares.) In the interest of the all-important bottom line, Big Food systematically tortures, drugs, and abuses meat animals, acting as if they weren't living beings at all, but mere products, like toasters or Tic Tacs. In so doing, they are not only behaving in a morally bankrupt fashion toward our fellow living beings, but they are putting the health and safety of the customers who ultimately will eat these animals at great risk as well—and that's us.

When the call finally came, I dropped everything and raced over to Randy and Annie's, afraid I'd arrive too late for the sending up of the final four. But I was right on time and Randy was calm, tired, and sweaty after a day that had started at six in the morning and wouldn't end till six that night. He wore a yellow rubber apron and giant black rubber boots and looked every bit the part of a man who'd been sending chickens to meet their maker all day, all for the sake of a healthy, sustainable diet for his family.

After drinking a tall glass of iced tea, he drove the tractor down to the coop where the chickens had lived the entirety of their ten-week lives. For only ten weeks old, they looked *enormous*: eight pounders most of them, with beady, wild eyes and muddy, reptilian, three-toed feet. One by one, Randy escorted the last four into the pull-behind trailer where—using his best black sense of humor to diffuse the tenor of the day—he had installed a handwritten sign reading: "Meet the Colonel

[meaning Colonel Sanders]—book signing today!" Then off
we drove to the killing cones.

Killing cones are a little like upside-down traffic cones,
except they are made of metal. They hang from a framework,
as does a flexible wire that is used to wrap the bird's feet, sub-
duing it and reducing struggling. The day was searingly hot,
and the flies buzzed about the blood that had already stained
the dirt underneath each cone. After Randy slit the throat
of the first bird, I was greatly relieved. I *could* do this with
no crying, no lost lunch, no fainting. Phew. I was astounded
to realize I was actually completely fine. Slowly, the blood
drained out of the bird, and you could almost pinpoint the
moment when the bird ceased its struggle and life simply
left—almost evaporated. It was perhaps the quietest, most
peaceful death a chicken could hope for, really.

Then Randy asked me something I hadn't expected: "Do
you want to do one?" *Oh.* Hmmm. Well…Why not? I mean,
who knows when I will ever get this chance again, right? And
that is how I came to be the last earthly friend of chicken
number 52.

The first time I slid the knife across its gnarly little neck,
I knew immediately it hadn't gone deep enough. Panicking,
and quite sure I was going to end up torturing and/or muti-
lating this poor creature, I quickly slid it again with greater
force, as if I were slicing a nice roast. This was better, if not
perfect, and the blood began to stream down the way I had
seen the other chickens' do. Hanging there in its aluminum
cone, it took only a minute or two to bleed out.

I wondered why I wasn't upset. I wondered if I should be
worried about the fact that I wasn't upset. (I'm a monster!
A conscious-less chicken murderer!) Meanwhile, Randy was

pulling the muddier feathers off the already deceased birds and laying them back in the pull-behind, while I watched number 52 intently. After some moderate flailing, he (she?) curled its head up suddenly in a question mark shape, staring directly at me (or so I thought). I imagined a quizzical look in its eyes that surely was not actually there and then—as if a switch had been flipped—its mouth yawned open at the same time as its neck relaxed; a white film came down over the chicken's beady eye. Even a neophyte like me could instantly recognize the aspect of death, and respect it, even in the small, awkward end of a chicken.

After Randy kills the chickens, there's still a fairly elaborate process to go through: he scalds them in 180-degree water (loosening the feathers), runs them through the feather picker (a Dead-Chicken Tilt-A-Whirl!), spinning the chicken bodies around in a rather startling, clumsy fashion while black rubber nodules remove most of the hard-to-pluck feathers. Then, on a carefully bleached counter, he eviscerates the bird, snipping off the head, feet, the scent gland above the tail, and then removing the internal organs one by one (intestines, liver, heart, windpipe, and lungs).

Once again, Randy let me try my hand at the procedure, and anyone who knows me pretty well will need to be revived after hearing that I eviscerated two still-warm bird bodies with Randy's helpful direction. I'm not sure why, but all my squeamishness disappeared. Perhaps it was the beginning-to-end nature of the process. Perhaps it was the fact that Randy helpfully talked me through each one, lung scraping and all. Perhaps I was just too fascinated by the fact that yes, each bird body was exactly the *same* on the inside! *Yup, there's the heart, right in the same place as the last one!* I was struck by the amazing predictability of biology. Is this how surgeons come to see people, I wondered, as different outwardly, perhaps, but basically just identical walking amalgamations of organs? "Yup, there's the heart, right in the same place as the last one."

I guess you end up thinking some odd things while pulling the organs out of a chicken.

Finally the bird is dunked in a spring-water bath to cool. Here they await the arrival of Annie on the scene to remove them from the bath, blot them inside and out with paper towels, and carefully wrap them for storage in the freezer. And you know what? It looks like chicken.

Fifty-two chickens, fifty-two weeks. Randy and Annie now had a freezer full of the finest-quality organic meat that will last them for an entire year. They knew where it came from. They knew what it had eaten, what it was treated like, and how it died. They had taken responsibility, on a very basic level, for their food.

Attending "processing day" surely isn't for everyone. But it was nice for me, at the very least, to spend and hour or two acknowledging where all that chicken we eat actually comes from—a silly, awkward animal, that still deserves our kindness and respect.

––––––––––

Of course, looking back over our food history, domesticated animals are only one part of the meat story. Since moving to Vermont, I've become much better acquainted with the most ancient kind of meat procurement: hunting.

Fortunately, the fact that I'm a meat eater now means that our family can look forward to enjoying the spoils of the hunt even though we *didn't* get up at the crack of dawn to go sit in a cold tree stand sprinkled with deer urine for several hours. Then again, who knows? At the rate we're going, maybe in another ten years we'll be doing that too.

If you had asked me to define "game supper" before I moved to Vermont fourteen years ago, I probably would've guessed a potluck involving Scrabble or possibly Bridge. At that time I was a confirmed "city mouse." To my mind the mention of "game" probably meant it was time to argue over who gets to be the top hat and who has to be the boot.

I can imagine how horrified *that* version of me would've been—the me who insisted that our sit-down wedding dinner for one hundred consist entirely of vegetables and fish—to encounter the annual festival of carnivorousness that is the Vermont Game Supper.

Every November (read: deer season), each town in our area has their own Game Supper benefitting deserving local causes such as the volunteer fire department and the sixth grade field trip. We had been to our local Game Supper for the last few years and the menu was reliable: Moose Meatballs (the whole reason to go), Bear Steak (to say you've had it), Chicken and Biscuits (for the very squeamish), and Venison, Venison, Venison. Venison Stew, Venison Steak, Venison Sausage, and if you're in luck, maybe Gib made his famous Venison Salami—only one piece per customer please, supplies are limited.

Of course there are sides too—mashed potatoes and squash—if you have any room left on your plate, which you won't. Salads, rolls, and paper plates filled with cocktail-size blocks of Vermont cheddar wait on the tables once you're done running the buffet line. And if you're *still* hungry— which you won't be—and still eating sugar (read: everyone except us), there's always the yawning expanse of the dessert table, with slices of apple, lemon merengue, and chocolate pie making kids drool from all the way over by the fire exit sign.

But the word on the street was, "Pssst! *Rupert's Game Supper is better.*" So this year we decided it was time to check that one out too. Why was Rupert's Game Supper better? Well, for one thing they used real dishes (not paper plates that sag under the weight of your Fred Flintstone-esque meal) *and* they can be counted on to have game even more unique than moose and bear. Which is how I came to try beaver. It's also how I came to spit beaver out into my napkin .0395 second later.

If anyone ever asks you to define what "gamey" tastes like, you should send them to try a nice dish of beaver. One friend remarked that eating beaver is like "eating an oil slick" and I have to say I couldn't agree more. But I *tried* it.

Another key difference between our town's and Rupert's suppers is that they wear funny hats at the Rupert Game Supper—antler headbands, chicken hats, sombreros, you name it. Nobody I asked knew why.

This year, however, I had a whole new appreciation for our Game Suppers as the one local event we could attend with confidence in our Year of No Sugar. The distinctions were crystal clear: the meat was on one side of the room, and the sugar was on the other. After all the back handsprings we'd done to ferret out fructose this year, the clarity of this division was quite comforting.

Which returns me to an increasingly familiar refrain: the idea of going back in time a bit in order to avoid the health impacts our over-processed, over-convenient life-style has bestowed upon us. There is a point at which all the hippy-dippy themes—no sugar, no plastics, no pesticides, eat local—start to converge; suddenly we begin to see what it is we've been driving at all along: what Great-Grandma used to cook. And much of it looked a lot like the Game Supper.

Although I'm pretty sure Great-Grandma never wore a funny hat.

————

One thing Great-Grandma *did* do that actually involved large quantities of sugar was make jam. Personally, I love to make jam. Every year I look forward to the various local harvests anticipating what interesting flavor I'll be able to concoct: peach-strawberry jam? Jalapeno pepper jelly? One year we ended up with a large bag of Italian plums that I cooked up, causing the entire house to smell of stewed prunes. *Oh no!* I thought. *Prune jam?* But in fact the *plum* jam was delicious.

But this year, of course, I had gone back and forth on the issue. To jam or not to jam? That was the question. Sure, jam was the kids' "exception food," so I could justify it on those grounds. But would I really be able to spend hours slaving over vats of boiling water and sterilized tongs only to *not* partake of the results myself? I wasn't sure I had willpower enough for that, so I held off.

It wasn't until September rolled around that the Concord grapes were weighing down my arbor with fragrant fruit that I decided I could stand it no more; I tried making a No-Sugar Grape Jelly. I had my work cut out for me. If you've never made jelly or jam, then you might be astounded to know exactly how much sugar is ordinarily devoted to the average batch; most jams contain more sugar than actual fruit—much more. It's not uncommon at all for a batch of, say, blueberry jam to call for seven cups of sugar. Yes. *Seven.* This works out roughly to a cup of sugar per pint jar. Think of *that* the next time you have toast.

And, like baking, jam isn't super improvisable. Unlike making a stew or omelet, where you can just throw in what you've got and get something edible at the end, jam is rather inconveniently science-y. In order to get jam or jelly to set up correctly, i.e., get that gelatinous, not-quite-liquid-not-quite-solid consistency, you have to have an appropriate amount of pectin, which naturally occurs in fruit and more so in unripe fruit. In the olden days, making jam must truly have been an art form: figuring out what percentage of ripe to unripe fruit to use, and after cooking, testing with a cold spoon to see if the jam had set properly, before beginning the long, hot procedure of boiling your sterile jars filled with jam to make them seal correctly for storage.

These days, most jelly and jam makers add powdered pectin to the cooking fruit, which ensures that your jam will set up like a golden retriever every time. In recent years, I've made many batches of delicious jam in just this way. So I wondered: What if I made a jelly that followed all the instructions but substituted *dextrose* for sugar? Would it work?

This was going to be a lonely journey, however. If you are a modern canner, then you know that the literature available about canning today is not for the faint of heart. "WHATEVER YOU DO," they all read in the most alarming font they can find, "DO NOT, REPEAT, <u>DO NOT</u> TAMPER WITH THESE RECIPES IN ANY WAY OR YOU AND EVERYONE YOU'VE EVER LOVED WILL MOST ASSUREDLY DIE FROM SOME TERRIBLE FLESH-EATING BACTERIA!!!!" I have at least four books with canning recipes, and they all say virtually the same thing: no improvisation allowed. NONE. Story's over, go to bed.

Meanwhile, if you talk to the old-timers, the ones who canned decades ago with crazy things like rubber seals and wax, you get an entirely different story. They all say the same thing: "Oh, it's *fine*. Don't worry. Jam is incredibly hard to spoil! And even if it does mold on the top a bit, you just scrape that bit off and eat it anyway." Now, I probably wouldn't go so far as to eat mold-encrusted jam, but wasn't there a happy medium we could arrive at here? Was a homemade no-sugar jam possible?

As I mentioned, the Concord grapevines in my backyard were sagging with fruit so I decided I would try my experiment on these. This added an extra step—I usually prefer jam with nice big chunks of fruit and skin throughout, but Concord grapes have to be made into jelly, not jam, because of the seeds and tough skins, which must be removed. After cooking and straining the grapes through cheesecloth, I began to boil the sweet juice.

Now right here I realized I already had a problem. Uh…juice? I stopped right in the middle of my steaming, pulp-slopped kitchen with the sudden realization. We haven't had *juice* since January 1, even as a sweetener. Year of No Sugar Rule #302: fruit must have corresponding fiber attached. Period. Huh. Why hadn't I thought of this before? What should I do? Well, I was dying to know if my experiment would work, and, I rationalized, if it did, it *could* be extrapolated to jams, which *would* include the skins and pulp. But today grapes were what I had to work with. So, onward.

Now, every box of pectin from the supermarket comes

with a long list of instructions for most types of jam or jelly you might want to make, so I dutifully followed the grape instructions to the letter: After discarding the seeds, skins, and pulp, I brought five and a half cups of my fresh Concord grape juice to a boil in a large open pot on the stove. This, by the way, is my favorite part of making jam or jelly—the incredible fresh cooking-fruit smell that permeates every corner of your home. Potpourri has nothing on this. If I were to invent a perfume, I think it might be Concord Grape No. 5 or quite possibly L'eau de Peach.

At this part of the procedure, with the boiling fruit in one pot and empty glass jars sterilizing surgically in another, I always feel like I'm engaged in some wonderful alchemical process that will transform some delicious but humble fruit into pure edible magic. They're so beautiful, jars of jam in translucent hues sitting glinting on our shelves, waiting to remind us in the depths of a Vermont winter what the tastes of summer were. In the case of our Concord grapes, it's even better because they're free: the things grow like weeds in our backyard, no matter how badly we treat them, but due to the seeds and skins, they aren't much of a tasty snack. Without the jelly, this wonderful taste would pretty much go to waste, enjoyed by our backyard birds alone.

So I followed the recipe. After boiling the intense, incredibly purple juice for ten minutes, I added a quarter cup of dextrose (instead of the called-for sugar) to a bowl containing the pectin powder and stirred this into the pot. (This is an extra step you do with what I buy, which is Low-Sugar Pectin; it enables you to use less sugar in your jam, say *five* cups of sugar instead of seven. Seriously.) Brought to a boil, I then added the rest of the dextrose—three and a half more cups—boiled it exactly one minute and then removed it from heat, and I began ladling into sterilized jars.

Actually, I cooked it longer than one minute, trying to ascertain whether the set-up would really occur using the dextrose. It *looked* right—gelatinous and jelly-ish. But I'd always relied on the alchemy of the pectin-sugar combination to do this part for me, so I was nervous. The boiling purple lava was ladled into the jars, hot lids screwed on "fingertip tight," and into the bigger pot they went for the final sterilization. The filled jars boiled underwater for the requisite five minutes before being pulled out with jar tongs to cool on a dish towel.

What do you want to hear first, the good news or the bad news? The bad news is that my jelly didn't set. The good news is that we proceeded to do what jelly and jam makers have done with failed jelly and jam since time immemorial: we had a lovely sauce. The kids liked it on crackers and on toast. It was sweet…ish. Unlike any jelly I'd had or made before, it truly tasted of the unalloyed grapes. Now, if only the set could be improved…

My research continued. I was determined to figure out what went wrong, and this was when I began to learn a lot of disturbing things. For one, guess what store-bought low-sugar pectin has *in* it? Now, if you can't guess by now, I'm going to be veeeeeeeery disappointed. Yes! SUGAR. That's right: the low-sugar pectin—"for use with less sugar!"—has *sugar* in it. How ironic. How totally predictable.

Turns out, there *is* a special pectin you can order or find at the health food store that contains *no* sugar, called Pomona's Universal Pectin. (Instead of being activated by sugar, it is instead activated by calcium.) Even Pomona's, however, doesn't list recipes entirely omitting sugar—honey, artificial sweetener, and juice concentrate are all listed, but no sign of the No Added Sugar recipe I'd been searching for.

Incidentally, I realized, language is very important here: it helps not to call it *jelly* or *jam*. *Fruit spread* seems to be the term of choice for No-Sugar variants of this process. Recipes are available online for fruit spread that look promising, although the ones I found don't allow for canning. Rather, they produce a batch that lives in the refrigerator or freezer, which is functional if not quite so beautiful—also probably retaining more nutrients. That might be worth a try.

But still, I wondered, was there some magical reason sugar was absolutely essential to canned jam and jelly? Was I going to kill my family with my homemade grape sauce? Why was the answer so strangely, incredibly elusive? Fortunately, a few credible resources do exist online to help those of us who wish to cross over to the dark side of messing with/understanding our canning recipes: both Oregon State and Colorado State Universities have good extension websites that finally helped explain what I wanted to know: that, yes, sugar acts not only as a flavoring agent, but *also* acts as a preservative. *And* it activates the pectin to activate the set.

Silly me, this meant I was adding pectin to my grapes without the required mountain-load of sugar present to *activate* it. Did putting it in my jelly do virtually nothing? Or would dextrose do the same job but just require different amounts? It seemed likely that my grape sauce would likely have a shorter shelf life than the average estimate of a year for canned items. I could live with that.

Wow. You'd think they'd cover all this in *Canning & Preserving for Dummies*, right? But they don't. Just shut up and follow the recipe, people. And anyway, what kind of crazy person would ever want to make grape jelly *without* sugar?

We were now getting beyond the tip of the iceberg as to what avoiding this one lousy ingredient really entailed. At the risk of repeating myself here (say it with me!), we *are* talking about a substance which our body has no need for and which we only began consuming in earnest in the short space of the last few decades, right? You have to ask yourself: should avoiding sugar *really* be this hard?

CHAPTER 15

HOLY FOOD

It was the end of November. Our family had gotten through a *lot* together: countless birthdays, Halloween, school picnics, Thanksgiving. It felt like we were coming into the home stretch and I think I was getting almost a little…complacent. I had managed to get through eleven months of blogging about my family, what we'd been eating—and not eating— and pretty much everything else incidental or important that had happened along the way. Consequently, I think I may have assumed there was nothing left that could surprise me. But you know what one big, huge, enormously large issue *hadn't* come up yet? Religion.

Religion and food have one quintessential thing in common: they are both topics one's philosophy can become so ensconced in that they dramatically affect everything else in your life. Which is to say, some people treat religion like their food, and some people treat their food like a religion. Perhaps the two were bound to meet—I just didn't expect that meeting to come in the form of a plastic bag of flyers hanging on my front door.

Inside this bag was a bunch of information about a local

church, just a few miles down the road from us, and an invitation to their services and Christmas play, as well as a DVD titled *The Case for Christ*. "Enjoy meaningful worship and music," it read in part. Well, that sounds good. It went on to detail community service, celebrating recovery…all positive things.

Then I got to the coupon for McDonald's. Stapled to it was a card that read "Come visit us on Sunday…Then go for a Sundae!" and quoted the Psalms "Taste and see that the Lord is good." I kid you not.

Is McDonald's proof that God exists? Apparently, some people think so.

I was speechless. The church endorsing fast food? Using junk food desserts as a reward for attending services? When I was a kid we survived the droning sermons and fourteen off-key verses of "Oh Thou Who Art Mine Antidisestablishmentarianism" by doodling on the offering envelopes and looking forward to the "fellowship hour" that followed. There, we knew, we could snag more refreshments than we were reasonably allowed while the grown-ups gabbed and drank coffee. That was crap food too, of course: butter cookies from supermarket tins and Kool-Aid. So then, was it *really* so different?

I would argue that it was different. What was different was that it was still *in* the church, designed to get members of the congregation to begin talking to one another, become friends, maybe even form a close-knit community that would support one another, all thanks to some free caffeine. Turning the local McDonald's into the honorary vestibule, to me, isn't quite the same.

Instead, this came off more as a cheap bribe. I wondered

about the technicalities: if you use the coupon without going to church, will you go to Hell? And if you go collect all your neighbors' coupons from their doorknobs before they get home, are you *definitely* going to Hell?

Back in Jesus's day, food was a simpler matter: some loaves, some fishes. Sugar as we know it had yet to be invented, likewise McDonald's. Honey is mentioned often in the Bible, usually as an indication of plentitude, as in "milk and honey." Back then the food symbol of ultimate sin? An apple.

Apples have since come a long way: a symbol in today's society of purity, wholesomeness, and nutrition, Snow White's experience notwithstanding. It does make me wonder though, if the Bible were written today, would Eve have offered Adam a sip of her McFlurry?

———

By way of avoiding that ever-present temptation represented by The World and Everything in It, we had become a little bit like Food Monks. And now, more than ever, the key to me seemed to be investing a *lot* of time making food. Pretty much, I was dividing my time between making food and writing about food…and if there was any time leftover, I did trivial stuff like pay bills, shower, brush teeth. At times it felt like I was emerging from being under the surface of a lake full of cultural assumptions about food. My head just above the surface of that water, I was only now opening my eyes and beginning to look around—it was amazing to me to begin to realize how very much time real food can take, and how good and satisfying that could feel.[62]

---

[62]And exhausting. Did I mention exhausting?

For example, one night I was making spaghetti and meat-balls, which sounds like a pretty simple thing. Once upon a time, I would've bought meatballs and sauce at the supermar-ket, and such a dinner would've taken about half an hour, tops. This time, however, it took up a not-insignificant portion of my day: in the morning I made bread—not only for our toast and sandwiches, but also as a meatball ingredient. I poured boiling water over oatmeal and let it sit an hour, then added more ingredients before kneading the dough and setting it in a bowl to rise. An hour later I came back to it, divided it into two loaf pans and let it rise some more. Half an hour after that I put them in the oven, and half an hour after that the bread emerged from the oven smelling like God.

Later in the day, after picking the kids up from school, it was time to make the sauce. After putting cans of diced and crushed tomatoes to stew in a pot with oil and garlic, I got out meatball ingredients—defrosted beef, grated Parmesan, measured spices—then mixed them all together with a paste made from the cut-up bread slices and water. After the sauce was finished reducing, it was time to form the mixture into meatballs and gently place them into the hot oil for frying. Each batch cooks in about ten minutes, and I fuss over them like a mother hen, trying to ensure they don't burn on one side or undercook on another—and most of all that they stay in one piece. Meanwhile, I put the water on to heat up for the spaghetti.

All this time Ilsa was "helping" by making a fruit con-coction composed of cut-up clementines and bananas. She had a name for it—I can't recall it exactly, but something like "Super Happy Loveliness"—and after an extremely long process of peeling and squeezing and sampling and mixing, she was inordinately proud of the end result she put on the dinner table.

I knew exactly how she felt.

I wondered: is it crazy to feel this way about food? Not eating sugar was a tremendous part of it—it was the reason for making my own bread and sauce after all—but that wasn't *all* of it. It was more than that.

Right around this time, I was reading *Into the Wild*, the true story of Chris McCandless (who went by the name Alexander Supertramp) and his journey to Alaska to attempt to be free from the trappings of society and live off the land, and his eventual death by starvation. Why was I reading *this*, I wondered, when I still have a stack of "homework" books to read dealing with sugar and nutrition? What did this have to do with A Year of No Sugar? Probably nothing.

But the answer came on page 167. Author Jon Krakauer relates that Alex had underlined a passage in Thoreau's *Walden* concerning "the morality of eating." I sat up and with wide eyes read what Alex had read:

> *It is hard to provide and cook so simple and clean a diet as will not offend the imagination; but this, I think, is to be fed when we feed the body; they should both sit down at the same table. Yet perhaps this may be done. The fruits eaten temperately need not make us ashamed of our appetites, nor interrupt the worthiest pursuits. But put an extra condiment on your dish, and it will poison you.*

Whoa. I stopped cold when I got to the "extra condiment" part. It jumped off the page at me as if it were printed in neon ink. Sure, he may be speaking metaphorically about that extra condiment being poison…but still. Didn't that *kind of* sound like he was talking about sugar? I was as fascinated by this passage as Alex was—Alex had written in the margins of his copy: "YES. Consciousness of food. Eat and cook with concentration…Holy Food."

As if this weren't enough, sometime after this, I was reading a magazine interview with spiritual philosopher Jacob Needleman,[63] who talked about the practice of "self-remembering" and "Conscious, willful attention to oneself…" So much of what we concern ourselves with in life is meaningless, he argues, whereas what most cultures describe as "God" has to do with what he calls "deep feeling." I wondered, was Alex looking for that "deep feeling" in the Alaskan wilderness? Is it possible—or am I just crazy here—to relate our search for God or "deep feeling" or whatever you want to call it to the practice of meaningful sustenance, what Alex called "Holy Food"?

Maybe I was way, way, waaaay out on a limb here, but we were within spitting distance of meeting our goal of a Year of No Sugar, and I was feeling philosophical. It somehow made sense to me to draw big, sweeping analogies between the modern-day cultural avoidance of real social contact in favor of reasonable facsimiles thereof—Facebook, Twitter, interactive video games—and our modern-day cultural avoidance of real, fulfilling nourishment in favor of reasonable facsimiles thereof—fast food, processed food, convenience food.

Is modern society based on our collective desire to run away from consciousness/deep feeling/God? Is it possible that a

---

[63]D. Patrick Miller, "Beyond Belief: Jacob Needleman on God without Religion," *The Sun*, December 2011, issue 432.

practice of what Alex called "Holy Food" could represent the fledgling beginnings of a way back to…what? Spirituality?

"…the imagination…I think, is to be fed when we feed the body; they should both sit down at the same table."

Yes, folks, it had been nearly a year into this journey and perhaps I had finally cracked: I had discovered the meaning of life in a bowl of spaghetti and meatballs.

CHAPTER 16

YOU'RE RUINING MY LIFE…MERRY CHRISTMAS!

L et me tell you—the whole Christmas in a No Sugar household business? It is *not* for the faint of heart.

The holidays were coming—and I mean this in the most ominous way possible. Sometimes it felt like we'd been in training for the month of December the entire year. Christmas, the mother of all sugar holidays, the most fructose-laden of them all—more than Thanksgiving (which is a limited, one-day-only gluttony); more than Halloween (which focuses almost exclusively on the kids); more than birthdays and Easter and Valentine's Day *combined*. As the dozens of mail-order catalogs arriving at our house every day clearly confirmed, Christmas, for many of us, is about celebrating the birth of Jesus through a month-long marathon of sweets, treats, cookies, and cake.

But that's not what bothered me. What bothered me was the dread that my children were expressing at the prospect of facing a sweet-restricted Christmas. Sure, we had discussed that Christmas itself would be the day we had our "special dessert" for the month, and that otherwise we would use dextrose to make versions of our favorite traditional treats…

but on this account my daughter Greta refused any and all attempts at consolation.

"OH help me…I feel so helpless, like I have no will or say in anything," she wrote in her journal one night. "Like my mom's & dad's say & will comes first and overpowers mine."

Oof.

Her entry went on to lay the blame for her situation on David Gillespie, from whom I'd derived so much inspiration. As we were getting ready for bed, I tried telling her that Mr. Gillespie was actually a very nice man, and I reminded her that he has six children of his own who also avoid fructose, including one daughter just her age. But Greta wasn't having any of it.

"I hate it! I hate it! I HATE IT!" she exploded, pounding her fists on her mattress. Her eyes were shining with tears.

OH help me. I'm totally bailing on the sugar project at Christmas. (I) mean you can't avoid Great Grandma Schaub's mincemeat cookies. Nor can you avoid Grandma Sharon's chocolate cookies & also Christmas cookies. I feel so helpless, like I have no will or say in anything. Like my mom's & dad's say & will comes first and overpowers mine. And like when Isaiah & Donovan (Greta's cousins) hear that we can't have sugar, they'll start stuffing their mouths with cookies, cake, and pie. And that frustrates me—can you understand that?

Sincerely
Greta

P.S. It's not Mom's fault, it's Mr. David Gillespie. And boy, I hate his guts. Every milligram of him.

—*from Greta's journal*

———————

Now, you'll recall that my oldest daughter does have a bit of a flair for the dramatic. But, believe it or not, this is by far the most displeasure she had expressed with our No-Sugar Year to date, and I have to admit, I was a bit taken aback. Of course, I hated the idea that "my" project was causing my children angst, sadness, ridicule at school...but I always *knew* there had to be that side of it, didn't I? Didn't I?

While Greta's outburst worried me, Ilsa worried me more. One chilly day, we were buying sandwiches at a local shop when she reached out her hand curiously to touch a bowl of something on the countertop near the coffee carafes. When Greta suddenly warned her, "That's *sugar*," Ilsa actually *flinched*.

Then one night, as she was cutting up a magazine for a craft project, Ilsa showed me an ad for Häagen-Dazs ice cream. "Mama, I'm glad we're not keeping this," she said. "It hurts me."

Oh. Shit.

"*Really*, honey?" I stopped what I was doing and looked at her closely.

"Yeah." She looked at me a little seriously, a little incredulously, as if to say, *What, you didn't* know?

SO...December was shaping up to a busy month around our house, what with me color-coding my pointy hat and broom collection and everything. Directly following the "I hate it" episode, I took a deeeeep breath and asked both girls to look at me from where they sat, half-tucked into their comforters in their parallel beds, each with its own coral reef of stuffed-animal life-forms.

"Listen," I said. "I want you to know. I know this year has been really, really hard. And I want you to know how much I appreciate the fact that you've gone along and done this project with me all year long. And it's almost over—the really strict part. It's *almost over*." I felt like a broken record, even though I meant it. Was there really nothing I could do to assuage this sadness/anger/pain I had willingly invoked in them? Would words—in which I put such complete faith—really fail me?

Then suddenly, as if on cue, Greta sat up and raised her index finger in the air, in a dramatic professor a-ha pose.

"My first biography!" she declared with an impish grin that had—at least for the moment—erased her tears. "My *T-e-r-r-ible* Childhood!"

I smiled. Now, *that* was more like it.

———————

But Christmas was still coming. And it just wouldn't be Christmas without cookies, would it? As much as hanging our stockings and running out of Scotch tape, *cookies* have become an intrinsic part of the way our culture celebrates the holiday season. Every family I know has their own unique and highly personalized cookie tradition.

When I was growing up, at our house it was jelly thumb-prints and chocolate chip meringues. Maybe this doesn't sound very Christmassy to you, but all I have to do is taste that buttery dough with a bit of raspberry jam, and I am instantly transported to the Christmases of my childhood. I have since realized that making those two cookies *together* also represented a thrifty way to not let any eggs go to waste:

thumbprints got the yolks, meringues the whites. In my husband's house it was—and still is—his mother's amazingly addictive sugar cookie cut-outs with icing and sprinkles. Every year the big green Tupperware bowl comes out and everyone knows what *that* means: Sharon's Christmas Cookies are not far behind. The famous family story about them involves Sharon making them far in advance one year, in an attempt to get ahead of the holiday mayhem, only to find that the boys had discovered her stash and eaten *all* the cookies in advance—perhaps also to get a jump on the holiday season.

Their punishment was that Christmas itself was, therefore, *cookie-less. Gasp!* Can you imagine such a thing?

As an adult, I learned from my cousin Gretchen that our family had a much older cookie tradition than what I had experienced as a child: a recipe that had been brought over from the old country called *flettin*. Every November, weeks before the holiday season really got under way, the family women used to convene and proceed to spend an entire day rolling, cutting, and frying dough. After being sprinkled with a mixture of powdered sugar and cinnamon, the delicate little things would be wrapped in linen and stored in the *attic* (!!) for several weeks to let them "age," which presumably made them more crunchy and crispy. I don't know about you, but I'm pretty sure in *my* house, the attic mice and bats would do a number on these cookie baskets similar to what my husband and his brother did to his mother's big green Tupperware bowl.

Nonetheless, in recent years, our family has revived the flettin tradition. It's a bit more of a production these days, since everyone is coming from all across New England rather than from down the block or across town, but all the planning pays off when we finally arrive at one of our houses and settle in to tie on the aprons. Even with the dough prepared in advance—a very strange recipe involving lots of sour cream, separated eggs, and kneading (who *kneads* cookie dough?)—it *still* takes pretty much all day. We always set up an assembly line with the flettin veterans at the fryers and novices and kids on cookie cutting and sugar-sprinkling detail.

For years, Gretchen had been threatening to send the story of our flettin tradition to the King Arthur Flour Company's magazine *The Baking Sheet*—with hopes they would finally resolve some of our long-standing debates: Has *anyone* else ever heard of this recipe? Do we *really* have to separate and whisk the egg whites, only to knead and pound the dough after their addition? And honestly, was that aging in the attic thing a *real* step, or yet another clever strategy for getting a head start on the holidays?

But Gretchen really did send our story in, and, amazingly, they published it in their 2011 holiday issue.[64] I loved the irony of me, toiling away on my No-Sugar blog while simultaneously appearing in a cooking magazine next to a gigantic mountain of sugary fried Christmas cookies.

But there's another irony here, I think. 'Cause you know what? Flettin are a *lot* of work, part of our family history, and a wonderful Christmas tradition, but psst…They're not THAT good. I mean, they're *good*. But is that really what we drive several hours for? What we slave over a hot fryer all afternoon for? "Linen in the attic" instructions notwithstanding, in my opinion, flettin always taste best *that* day, warm from the fryer, freshly sprinkled and eaten while surrounded

---

[64]Susan Reid, "Baking Across America," *The Baking Sheet*, vol. XXII No. 6 Holiday 2011, page 12-13.

by family, some of whom you won't have the opportunity to see again till we do this *next* year. We don't have much in the way of family heritage, so Gretchen and I are holding on to flettin tight; it's not really about the cookies as much as about the fact that they're *our* cookies.

As it turns out, this year the family *didn't* manage to get together for a flettin day, so I didn't have to confront what it would mean in light of No Sugar—too bad. I was kind of looking forward to attempting a dextrose batch, and I felt pretty sure my family would've humored me, although they've been balking at my suggestion to replace the frying Crisco with lard, the way our ancestors would've surely fried flettin prior to the invention of hydrogenated oil in 1911.

Instead, I contented myself creating some oxymoronic recipes at home such as No-Sugar Sugar Cookies and Dextrose Gingerbread. They were getting good reviews from my helpers and harshest critics—the kids. Thus, despite all our fretting, I had a sneaking suspicion that a No-Sugar Christmas might just work out fine.

Later on, I wouldn't be so sure.

———

Grandma Sharon's Christmas Cookies were going to be our final treat for the year—it was one more thing we just couldn't imagine going without. We arrived at Grandma's after the compulsory marathon drive to get there—exhausted and feeling like sardines freed from our tin—and *there it was* on the kitchen counter: the big green Tupperware bowl. We didn't even have to look. We knew it was filled with frosted, sprinkled cookies in shapes of Santa and Christmas trees.

The fact that Sharon had been ultra-efficient as usual

presented a bit of a problem for me, however, one that I hadn't anticipated: we weren't going to be eating Christmas cookies all week; we could only have them on one day, for one dessert. How were we going to stare at that bowl *all week*, knowing those cookies were inside it? Ack! Was this some new form of torture?

Additionally, Sharon likes a sweet now and again, so a blue glass bowl of Hershey's kisses or hard candies is an ever-present fixture on her counter. On top of that, add the myriad treats that inevitably appear as presents or hostess gifts this time of year, not to mention the more ordinary stuff: there was juice in the fridge, ice cream in the freezer—hey, this *wasn't our house!* I knew my mother-in-law wasn't *trying* to torture us with things we couldn't have—after all, she had jumped through flaming hoops trying to find a Christmas Day ham that contained no sugar glaze of any kind. (All to no avail, as it turns out. Such a thing as an unglazed holiday ham in December is rarer than plaid shorts at a motorcycle rally.)

I knew Sharon probably thought we were crazy—make that definitely thought it—and that she had ever so politely refrained from actually saying so out loud, which I appreciated. But I was pretty sure that I was being paranoid that she was actually taunting us with that bowl of Hershey's Kisses. After all, that bowl was *always* there. And Greta and Ilsa weren't the only grandkids. It just *wasn't our house*.

Right?

We were in the home stretch, which may have been the sole thing that saved us. We toughed it out. We sucked it up. We knew in a few days Christmas would bring for us not only a visit from old St. Nick, but also a visit from the Christmas Cookie Fairy, and then it would only be a few more days until our year, *The* Year, The Year of Mommy Using Up Her Lifetime Quotient of Unreasonable Requests would be officially over. We were *so close.*

Maybe I should've known Aunt Carol's house would be the hardest of all. Why? Because Aunt Carol is great. She is the kind of relative who not only bakes fourteen different kinds of cookies for the holidays, but also bakes enough to give every relative who's in town a huge sampler plate of them to take home as well. She's been known to make her own chocolates and to decorate kids' birthday cakes so elaborately they might do for a medium-size wedding reception.

I identify with Aunt Carol in this respect: food is an expression of love. And up until this year, I too brought a sweet gift for all the relatives that I had made in my kitchen. Some years I brought homemade jams, others I made little cakes. In the years when our kids were really small and making something myself wasn't happening, I brought locally made gifts, like maple-sugar cotton candy and maple cream spread. Sensing a theme here? If food can equal love, then I guess sugar can equal Christmas.

As I mentioned, this year we were spending the holidays in Michigan with my husband's extended family, as we do every alternate year. A good eleven-hour drive from home, the area is a suburban ocean between the city-shores of Toledo and Detroit, and there's just a lot more of *everything* there: people, convenience stores, fast food restaurants, chain restaurants, billboards, freeways, parking lots, sirens, you name it. And it's not just the negative stuff. There's more variety there too: we can't get authentic Greek or Lebanese or Indian food in Vermont, but we can get it there. Coming from our little

Vermont town of a thousand residents, the sheer contrast can create cultural whiplash.

But back to Aunt Carol. Since long before I ever happened upon the scene, my husband's family has been getting together to exchange gifts on Christmas Eve. This year, Aunt Carol had volunteered to host, so we all arrived in our Christmas coats and fancy shoes at 6:05 on the dot.

Immediately, it was a *problem*. Greta took one look at the usual spread—cookies on the counter, fudge in a pretty glass basket, local Dietsch's chocolate samplers open on the sideboard—and quickly came to the conclusion that this was going to be the *worst Christmas ever*.

Ilsa, by comparison, was easy. She asked, "Can I have this?" and when the inevitable answer was no, she shrugged and ran off to go play. It may be that Greta just has a bigger sweet tooth, but I think the more likely possibility is that she has a preteenager's burgeoning need for independence and to make her feelings known by all in the immediate vicinity. She, unlike Ilsa, spent a good portion of her Christmas Eve pouting and making meaningful, tragic faces in my direction.

Dinner wasn't much easier. As she has other years, Aunt Carol had lovingly and graciously provided a buffet for all of us, and, ungrateful wretches that we were, we couldn't eat most of it. There was store-bought pulled pork and chicken, white and whole-wheat buns, baked beans, applesauce…Of course, sugar, to one degree or another, was in *all* of it. I don't know if it was intended for our benefit, but I was extremely, deeply grateful for the one large tray of mac and cheese that evening. If not for that, we would've been stuck eating olives for dinner, and I'm pretty sure Greta would've gotten enough mileage out of that to extend her extreme pout fest well into her thirties.

None of the relatives said much about the Sugar Project, probably because they think I'm loopier than the Cocoa Puffs bird for talking my family into it in the first place. But they all were as nice as ever, asking us all about the drive and Vermont and exclaiming about how the kids have grown, so I figured they still liked me anyway.

And then, thankfully, the present opening began. Greta and Ilsa were fully diverted for the remainder of the evening opening gifts, trying things on, helping the babies and toddlers, and creating a Bionicle masterpiece with cousin Donovan. That sour, Grinchy frown disappeared from Greta's face, and it was replaced by the happiness of being a kid at Christmas. Thank God.

Granted, having Greta's dining seat right next to a plate of forbidden chocolates and cookies on Christmas Eve wasn't ideal. But it was, I think, the biggest challenge we had had all year, and we survived it. I was proud of that—and proud of my family. And profoundly grateful for them. A good way to feel on Christmas, I think.

So what did *I* bring as gifts this year? Sweet things from my kitchen, of course! Over the prior few weeks I had been experimenting with quick breads of all kinds—banana, apple, pumpkin pecan, all made with no fructose, just fruit and good old dextrose—all tied up with a pretty little bow.

When the big day finally came and all the Christmas presents had been opened and scattered everywhere, it was time to caravan over to Sharon's fiancé's house for the kind of buffet meal that I think is so much fun on holidays: everyone is milling around—children, toddlers, grown-ups—picking at the vegetable plate and spilling juice and exclaiming about the quality of the roast beef. There's always a football game or an Indiana Jones movie on the television, and someone always leans back in the recliner and looks as if they may just fall asleep amid all the celebratory hubbub and everything.

It was amid this pleasant disorder that I snuck over to Sharon's Christmas Cookie plate, displayed next to a rainbow of store pies on the sideboard. It felt odd, because throughout the year we'd always had our monthly desserts as a family, as in "all for one and one for all!" But by the very nature of this particular event, that kind of solidarity wasn't happening—my family was happily spread all over the house. Nonetheless, I wasn't going to miss our final treat, our twelfth official added-fructose-containing item of the last 365 days, and I *sure* wasn't going to wait until all Sharon's famous cookies had been eaten. I carefully picked up a particularly thick-looking Santa cookie and considered it. I brought it to my mouth and then bit it.

Yes, I thought, *there it is.* That buttery, almost cakey cookie topped with thin, cool frosting and that hint of crunchy sprinkles almost an afterthought. There it is.

Do you remember the end of *The Grinch Who Stole Christmas*, when the Grinch pauses and is amazed to realize that Christmas has still come to the Whos, even though he has stolen all their presents? Sure, my one and only Christmas cookie was good. So good. But, we must ask ourselves, how good can a Christmas cookie be? Good enough to *be* Christmas?

I was as amazed as the Grinch to realize, just at that particular moment, that Christmas had come…*without* any fructose at all. It came!

Somehow or other it came, just the same.

CHAPTER 17

SUGAR AT MIDNIGHT

Ilsa is young enough that she still uses a handful of words she hasn't realized yet that she herself made up. One of them is *gladfully*, which she uses to mean "thank goodness," as in: "We arrived just in time for the movie, *gladfully*."

There's something inspiring about that to me, about the fact that she assembled that word one day, out of necessity to express a particular emotion and drawing from all her previous experiences. And it worked, so here she is still using it. When we're kids, we're much more used to figuring stuff out, to winging it. By necessity, kids are improvising all the time. As Indiana Jones once famously said, in the middle of some superhuman feat or other, "I don't know! I'm making this up as I go."

This year, we were making it up as we went too. As we approached New Year's Eve, I was quite stunned to realize that we were truly on the precipice of being through with our entire yearlong project. I felt as if I had been pedaling a fourteen-wheeled bicycle that had required my complete and total concentration for miles and miles, only to suddenly look up and realize I was within three feet of the finish line.

AAAA!! Oh no, I just can't think what life is going to be like after the project is done?? Well, we've all sort of evolved or should I say adapted. Adapted to the point it's like we're mutants. I just don't know what to think??!!… The point is…well, the point is ugh…OK fine, I'm scared of eating sugar again.

Isn't it weird how I don't know how to react to this? And I know and have known for the past few months (since mid-September) that this project has changed my whole entire life. And which is it positive or negative I really don't know?? So you see I'm very confused. VERY CONFUSED!!!!!

Help—Greta

—from Greta's journal

Looking back to the very beginning of our year, I was impressed by how awfully clueless we had been about what A Year of No Sugar would entail: we had yet to fully understand what fructose was, its many, many aliases, and what the deal was with omnipresent "no sugar" ingredients like sugar substitutes and sugar alcohols. I had yet to go through my banana, date, coconut, oligofructose, and "what do you *mean* I can't have carob?" phases. I had yet to read David Gillespie's *Sweet Poison* and through it to discover dextrose as a non-fructose sweetener. All I knew was that Dr. Robert Lustig's YouTube lecture had convinced me: sugar was a toxin. Poison.

Now, as we sat on the verge of being done with our No-Sugar Year, I felt a crazy mix of emotions: relief, delight, surprise, apprehension. Even though New Year's is traditionally associated with new beginnings, in this case it was also a definitive ending. I wondered: What would happen next? What was it all for? Had we changed our lifestyle for the better, or had we merely stubbornly proved a point? I took offense when a friend termed our project an "intellectual exercise," as if that characterization somehow minimized our effort—but *did* it? And was it? Perhaps the answers to those questions would be slowly revealed to us as we progressed forward into our next year: the Year of Figuring Out What To Do Now.

In preparation for the official end of our year's project, we'd had a whole series of family conversations about this what-happens-next business, and a lot of talk had centered around looking forward to things we hadn't been able to enjoy this year. One morning, I took a breakfast table poll and found out that Greta missed BLTs as much as anything, and that Steve missed restaurant condiments even more than dessert: ketchup on his French fries, salad dressing on his salad, mayo on his sandwiches. After careful consideration, Ilsa decided that, in addition to maple syrup, she was looking forward to having Jell-O (which is kind of funny since we *never* make Jell-O).

Me? I missed a good chocolate chip cookie, for which we never did find a suitable fructose-free replacement. If we ever make it back to Italy, even if it's in February, I intend to have more than one gelato. I was looking forward to being able to eat out without giving our waitress the Spanish Inquisition.

It's safe to say that Steve was especially excited about the end of our No-Sugar Year. I knew this because, during our Christmas travels, he bought a handful of Dutch chocolate bars and a sixty-four-piece Lebanese pastry sampler for us to enjoy "after the first." I was trying not to be alarmed about this mild case of gourmet sugar hoarding—after all, how many husbands would've been supportive of a family project like this one? Then, one night when I expressed a lack of interest in a sugared dessert, Steve made the comment, "*Hey*—I want my wife back." I must admit, this kind of freaked me out. Back? Had I gone somewhere? Was I no longer the person who loved a good Reese's Peanut Butter Cup? Had I become a permanent killjoy?

I didn't think so—at least I hoped not. The way I saw it, it was quite the opposite: my appreciation for food and where it comes from, what it's made of, and what is required for its preparation had gone up manifold. More than anything, our no-sugar year had taught me how much I *love* food, how important it is, and how little attention our culture collectively pays to it. Food is the stuff of life—we are what we eat—feeding yourself well is caring for yourself—choose your favorite adage. It's all truer than we could ever fully realize.

This year had taught me that, just like anything toxic—alcohol, nicotine—we need as a society to start handling sugar (fructose) with care, as potentially addictive, potentially dangerous. I wondered, Can we even *do* that? Do we have the self-possession to realize that "moderation" does not mean "whatever the amount *I* eat is"?

I had come to understand that sugar, while fun, is nutritionally expensive. Why would I want to waste my allotment of it on vending machine cookies or breakfast cereal? Why not save it for that something truly special? Americans instead simply decide to have it all—the good, the bad, and the ugly—and then are tragically surprised when health ramifications ensue. No one ever told them sugar could be really, truly harmful.

But what *would* happen after January first? I disliked the chaos of not knowing. After a year of rules, I was desperately groping for guidelines. Consequently, as we approached New Year's Eve, my new year's proposal to my family was to have dessert with actual sugar in it once per week. After this year, that sounded to me like a whole lot, but then again, after our adventures at Christmas visiting relatives and friends, being reminded how much sugar is involved in the average American's everyday life, I thought it was a reasonable compromise.

Likewise, in the new year we planned to return to eating bacon and ketchup without fear. We'd buy Hellman's Mayonnaise again for our tuna fish sandwiches. I wouldn't blanch at restaurant bread that had a teaspoon of sugar in the ingredients. Heck, I might even stop taking cell phone pictures of my food.

No promises though.

Some things, however, would stay permanently changed. Juice would remain off the table; soda always was.[65] I almost never bought box cookies or other store-bought desserts before; moving forward, those would be promoted to the "never ever" list. I would continue to check my crackers and other products, avoiding anything with sugar as a filler ingredient. Fast food restaurants were still entirely out. Chain restaurants would be in the category of "in case of extreme and most desperate emergency." Instead of them, we'd stubbornly continue to seek out good restaurants, local restaurants, places where they actually *make* the food they serve. At home, I would continue to make my own pizza, tortillas, yeasted

---

[65]Well, for everyone in our house except Steve that is. Anyone know the hotline number for Diet Dr Pepper Anonymous?

breads, and quick breads. Perhaps most significantly, I would continue to use dextrose for everyday baking and cooking.

Was I worried about going forward with the rules changing in this fashion? Nervous we'd go overboard like an alcoholic who thinks he's got his act together and can handle it? I was. But Steve likened our No-Sugar Year to what he experienced in the Marines. "You go through an experience that changes you," he says, "and you get out and you say, 'Now what?' But still, you really aren't the same. That conditioning is always there. That's how I feel."

I honestly didn't expect us to plow through those Lebanese pastries in the same fashion as we would've a year ago. Rather, I imagined we'd have a bite or two—as we each did with our allotment of sugar cookies on Christmas Day—and then say, "That's good. And *sweet*!" And it would be enough.

And so, at midnight, as we watched Lady Gaga blather on the TV about how magical New Year's is in New York City, we each ate our personally selected treat for the evening (Ilsa: a cookie, Steve and Greta: a Lebanese pastry, me: a Reese's Peanut Butter Cup). A lot of friends and family had focused on this New Year's Eve moment as if it were absolutely pivotal: the freeing of the taste buds from bondage! It was inevitably a little anticlimactic. For me, the next morning was the real question mark. What would the legacy of our year *really* be?

Only time would tell. Gladfully.

———————

Pop quiz: What's harder than a Year of No Sugar?

Answer: The week *after* a Year of No Sugar.

Oy vey. I wondered why on earth I had ever, *ever* looked forward to our release from the world of No Sugar. Our first week out of the project was easily as hard as our very hardest No-Sugar week. Why? Because, while No Sugar may be hard in terms of willpower, once we learned all the synonyms and safe words, it was always extremely clear in terms of the rules: "No Sugar" means: No. Sugar.

No sugar in our mayonnaise. No sugar in our bacon. Not in buns or salad dressing or juice. I will not eat it in the house. I will not eat it with a mouse. Everywhere we went well-meaning waitresses and relatives and friends would politely try to argue "but there's only a *little*...look! It says .00001%!" But the rules as we had made them were simple. "Is it in the ingredients?" I would ask. And of course, it always was.

I loved the straightforwardness of that. And I was hating the lack of it now.

For breakfast New Year's Day, we decided to visit one of our favorite local restaurants, Rathbun's Maple Sugar House. The last time we had been there had been a million, billion years ago: *last* New Year's Day, the very first day of our No-Sugar family experiment and before I was fully understanding that a pancake house would be entirely off the table in such a project. (Once again, Eve being a little slow on the uptake.)

Immediately, the questions started coming. "Can we get a hot chocolate?" "Can we have maple syrup?" "Can we have *juice*?" No hot chocolate. Yes maple syrup—but not a lot. No juice.

And the questions just kept coming. I certainly couldn't blame the kids—they were simply trying to figure out what the new rules were. Trouble is, Steve and I didn't exactly know. *Moderation* is the most elusive term I know.

A morning not long after that, Steve made another favorite and long-forbidden treat: crepes with sugar and butter.

Oh, how we had missed those. Sure, it was a lot *less* sugar than he would've ever used before, but I was starting to feel anxious. To me, it felt like things were spiraling out of control. It was January, so of course it was Ilsa's birthday again, and then it was my mother's birthday, and then we had the kid party for Ilsa's birthday...It was starting to feel like sugar was creeping its way back like a virus—between the long-lost condiments, the "remember this's," and the birthday treats. It suddenly seemed like sugar was absolutely freakin' everywhere. After all we had gone through over the course of the past year, I was struck now by the paralyzing thought: *Had it all been for* nothing?

And then I took the girls to the supermarket. "*Mom!* Can we buy these crackers? And cereal? Actual *real* cereal?" "Ooo! What about *roast beef?*"[66] It reminded me of that scene in *Moscow on the Hudson* in which Robin Williams plays a Russian defecting to the United States. He enters an American supermarket for the first time in search of a can of coffee and, confronted with an entire aisle, floor to ceiling, of different styles, brands, sizes, promptly faints. Choice is good but too much choice? It can be *bad*. Gritting my teeth, I capitulated on the crackers, but demurred on the cereal and roast beef. One thing at a time, I said.

I had even promised them—in a fit of guilt for all my family had put up with in the last year—to get them each a small check-out counter treat on the way out, as we had used to do quite often in the old days. This simple task, it turns out, was a fiasco. Did you know that ALL gum these days has not just sugar in it, but *also* sugar alcohols (maltitol, sorbitol,

---

[66]Remember, most supermarket cold cuts have sugar-containing glazes in them.

xylitol) or aspartame, and that most of them have *both*? We were unable to find a single package of gum in which sugar was the *only* toxin. So I did something I hate to do: I broke my promise.

I was astounded. After months of swerving to avoid processed foods, I was confronted once again with the ugly reality. Do we really give this little of a shit about what we're putting into our bodies, our kids' bodies? I thought back to the huge sacks of Halloween candy the kids had brought home in October—I mean, who *knows* what was in all that stuff. (Thank God it all still sits uneaten in the back of our pantry cupboard. My new plan is to throw it away after they've both gone to college.)

Aside from making us sound like we were from planet Pluto when we went shopping at the supermarket, another immediate and interesting by-product of our No-Sugar Year was that I now *really* noticed what sugar was doing in my body after I ate it. When I ate a cookie or had a piece of chocolate, here is what happened: I realized that after a moment my mouth felt...*funny*: cloying and overly sweet, like I just drank a whole glass of maple syrup. A few minutes would pass, and I'd feel a small headache-y feeling creeping around the base of my brain, followed by a weird energized feeling, a sugar "buzz" if you will. After a while, of course, it passed.

You'll recall that *Sweet Poison* author David Gillespie had written that after a while, you "just don't want" the taste of sugar anymore. During our entire Year of No Sugar, I found I never quite arrived at that train station. I kept *wanting* things. Sure, over time I wanted them *less*—the voice in my head wasn't so much a yell anymore as it was kind of whispery whine—but I never felt the wanting disappear *entirely*. On

Day 364, did I still *want* the croissants at our favorite bakery, an ice cream cone on a hot day, ketchup on our French fries? Yes. Yes, I did.

But now what struck me perhaps most of all was the fact that when I would give in and have a something that I wanted, or *thought* I wanted, or somebody else thought I should want, often it failed to be enjoyable at all. This was newly noticeable—a disconnect between what my brain thought I'd enjoy and what my body actually *did* enjoy.

For example, one day at a fundraising event, the girls came back from the refreshment table with—no, not the plates of grapes and cheese they were selling—a dense hunk of chocolate chip cookie dough covered in chocolate (Greta) and an iced cookie the size of a small salad plate (Ilsa). I thought, *Have they learned* nothing *this year!?!* But then again, who was I to blame them for wanting to partake, to enjoy, after an entire year of hanging back and repeatedly saying "no, thank you"? At this point, they knew more about sugar than most grown-ups we knew. Sooner or later, I'd have to take the gloves off and let them make some of these decisions on their own.

Interestingly, Greta absolutely *insisted* on giving me half of her "cookie dough truffle," which, not so very long ago, she would've had to elbow me out of the way to get (cookie dough *anything*? I'm so there!). So I took a bite of it—and immediately I was confused. I knew I was *supposed* to like it. All my senses were telling me I *would* like it—the texture, the smell, the appearance—and yet…I didn't. I just didn't. It was sickly sweet and left a bad aftertaste lingering on my tongue. Once upon a time, I would've had a hard time not going back for two or ten more of these funky little concoctions. Now? I was pretending to enjoy it. I was relieved when it was gone.

So, was this weird yet? I realized it wasn't just for my family's benefit that I was pretending to enjoy things that I once would have loved. It was also me trying to fool myself into thinking I was no different than I once was. But I *was* different. I wondered how long this would last—would I *ever* enjoy sugar again? Or had I inadvertently removed all the joy of sweet from my life? Given myself a taste bud-ectomy? For all my thousands of hours writing and researching about the evils of added sugar, I couldn't help but admit that in the end, I felt quite ambivalent about that. Did this mean no more homemade rhubarb pie? No more afternoons canning sour cherry jam? No more (and I hesitate even to type these words) *chocolate peanut butter ice cream*? Picking cherries, making pie from rhubarb just picked in our yard, all these things are rituals which have come to define, in some ways, who I am. Heck, I ate a chocolate peanut butter ice cream cone the night before *each* of my two girls were born. (Now there's a selling point for Ben & Jerry's: It's cool! It's delicious! And it may induce labor!)

So, for those of you keeping score at home, the aftermath of our Year of No Sugar consisted of me being plagued by fears that:

a. We would go right back to where we had started—all sugar, all the time.
b. We (I) would never *really* enjoy sugar again.

Notice anything a little funny about that? Apparently, I was simultaneously worried that we'd be eating both too much sugar *and* not enough. I wish I had saved myself the angst, but I suppose that me being a neurotic mess at first was kind of inevitable. After all, I had been possessed, obsessed by the idea of A Year of No Sugar, but I hadn't had any epiphanies on what to do *after* the Year of No Sugar. So instead, I fell apart.

Steve, who deserves the Golden Husband Award for going along with No Sugar in the first place, was more ready than I was for life to go back to normal. As in: We did it! It's over. This difference in our attitudes about moving forward was brought into sharp focus one day at lunch.

It all started when I, deep in the throes of sugar paranoia, asked Steve *not* to buy a new container of maple syrup. This segued into whether I'd continue to bake with dextrose and touched on things like whether banana bread and apple muffins count as dessert and whether snacking between meals is okay. I imagine some people would think we were giving what we eat and how we eat it entirely too much thought, bordering on obsessive, and maybe we were. I really didn't know anymore. It was exhausting. Personally, right then, I was feeling like moderation kind of sucked—it took entirely too much thought and energy, not to mention fighting. I was pretty sure it would be preferable to go live under a tree stump and only eat pinecones from now on.

Of course, we can't do that. And I honestly had no desire to be the dietary freaks of our community who carry their own marinated sawdust or whatever in a pouch with them so they can eat separately but equally everywhere they go—no. Yes, I admire folks like Scott and Helen Nearing or Tasha Tudor for being so passionate about their unique ways of life—they are fascinating to me. But their sacrifices were huge: these are folks who had to remove themselves from society to follow their ideals—which, above all, sounds pretty lonely.

Not long after that discussion, we had a babysitter night, so Steve and I went out to try a new restaurant. At the end of a nice meal, Steve became convinced I wanted dessert. A year ago, I wouldn't have even considered it a proper meal out without that final sweet component, but this time I demurred. I was full. I didn't want any. Still, he kept encouraging me to pick something from the menu. There was no convincing him that I didn't, in my heart of hearts, *want* the chocolate chip cookie sundae but—much to my astonishment—I didn't. I mean, I *really* didn't!

All that month, I'd been playing guilty catch-up from a year of denial, with my kids, with my husband, with myself. It was pretty hard to say no now, after my family had given sugar up for a year, on my say-so. Because I thought it was a good idea. Because I thought it would make us healthier. Because I wanted to write about it.

So I didn't say no as much as I wanted to right then. Selfishly, I didn't want my kids to think I'd become the Scrooge of the food universe, or my husband to think he's lost his fun wife who used to get all giddy at the thought of combining chocolate and peanut butter. I still do, after all. I'm still fun. Right?

Right?

So did we order the ridiculously sinful chocolate chip cookie in a cast-iron pan with ice cream and whipped cream on top? Sure we did, because I'm still fun, damn it. I was almost embarrassed by the conspicuous decadence of the thing when it arrived; I felt as if we had a circus elephant sitting on our table. I had a few bites and of course it was very good—in the way that only a warm cookie with cold ice cream on it can be. Very good. But then I put my fork down. I was happy to see that really, *really*, I could take it or leave it.

––––––––––

The reactions to the end of our project from friends, acquaintances, and readers were fascinating to me. Many people said "Congratulations!" which is lovely, and many more seemed simply relieved that we aren't doing "that sugar thing" anymore, just in case it might rub off on them or something. Half the people I encountered seemed to expect us to now be on a permanent sugar binge in order to make up for lost time, while the other half seem to think we're terrible hypocrites if we so much as glance at the bowl of mints by the restaurant door.

The fact is, for us, it was ever so much more complicated than "All Sugar All the Time!" or "No Sugar Never Ever!" My kids still wanted to get a dish of ice cream after dinner the way they always did. And me—selfish, guilty parent that I am—I often really wanted to give them that dish of ice cream as if it were a nice, compact serving of normality I could hand them with a pretty cherry on top. "See!? We're not so weird after all!"

But, the thing is, we *are* weird. We were weird *before*—not eating at McDonald's and avoiding soda. And we're weird *now*—avoiding juice and crap sugar food (doughnuts, cookies, free lollipops), as well as anything that's sweetened when we know it needn't be: dried fruit, chips, crackers, tomato sauces. We had become much, *much* more selective about the sugar we do consume, and in a culture like ours—which is utterly saturated with sugar, convenience food, and fast food—that's *weird*.

Then again, we were much more mainstream than we were *last* year. We had stopped flipping out about things like orange juice in the salad dressing or sugar in the bread. We were no longer the most annoying table our waitperson had that night, which was nice for everybody. And anyway, after a year of questions, we also already *knew* which items would have the sugar in them. Sometimes we had them, and sometimes we didn't.

But after inoculating myself with small amounts of sugar on a regular basis—a teaspoon's worth here and there—I had found that gradually, over time, my ability to enjoy sugar—without aftertaste or headache—had returned. It was different, though. I now enjoyed things with a much, much subtler sweetness than I ever would've thought possible. Sodas, ice cream sundaes, carnival cotton candy all now strike me as slightly…gross. However, I *can* order the mango sticky rice at the Thai place and simply *enjoy* it.

Which I view as a good thing. After all, alcohol is a potentially addictive poison, but that doesn't stop me from enjoying a glass of it with dinner on a regular basis. Likewise, I want to be able to enjoy a bit of fructose—potentially addictive poison anyone?—in the occasional dessert. For me, that's part of the joy of life.

So I'll have my glass of wine and maybe a small dish of the amazing gelato at that Italian restaurant. But I'm walking right by ninety percent of what's for sale at my local supermarket—row after row of sugar-sweetened beverages, snacks, candy, and convenience entrees. We drink water, snack on whole fruit, rudely ignore candy, and cook from scratch. It's not as simple as "Yes, always!" or "No, never!" but that's fair, I guess. Food is what keeps us alive, brings us together every day, and gives us the means to celebrate and enjoy. If that isn't worth our serious consideration, I don't know what is.

THE MORAL OF OUR STORY

One who is full loathes honey from the comb,
but to the hungry even what is bitter tastes sweet.

Proverbs 27:7

If I've heard it once, I've heard it a thousand times. It's the story of my grandfather and the grapefruit.

Because my father's father died when I was about ten years old, and because he lived far away in California, I don't have very many memories of him. Instead, much of what I know of my grandfather comes from stories others have told me, and the story I have heard the most is the one told by my mother.

It goes like this: my mother, a young bride, sat at the table with her husband's family and politely asked to have the sugar passed so she could sprinkle some on her grapefruit. My grandfather, being the very opinionated guy that he was, proceeded to give her a lecture on why grapefruit was perfectly palatable as nature intended it to be without requiring adulteration.

Because, by all accounts, he was a pretty headstrong guy, he seems to have phrased this in a rather undiplomatic manner, something along the lines of "Only a complete *moron* would add sugar to a perfectly good grapefruit!" Or something like that.

I'm not positive, but I'm pretty sure at the time that my mother was cowed into submission and resentfully ate her grapefruit plain, casting sidelong annoyed glances at Mr. Self-Appointed-Dietary-Dictator all the while. But then again, maybe not. Maybe she defiantly sprinkled her sugar, adding an extra pinch for good measure just to show *him*.

I don't really know, because for my mother that was beside the point. The point of the story was this: her new father-in-law was telling her what to do—specifically *how to eat*, as if there was a correct way and an incorrect way to go about the matter. And she certainly did not like it. No, she did *not*. Did he deter her from adding sugar to her grapefruit in the interest of *not* being a moron? Hardly. My mother sugars her grapefruit with enthusiasm to this very day, and I'd daresay she thinks of John Ogden every single time she does it.

This, then, is our conundrum. How do we attempt to come back from the brink of disaster, emerge from the out-of-control obesity epidemic that threatens to swallow our population whole? Dr. Robert Lustig likened the Candyland of modern western culture to an opium den. So how do we begin to emerge from that opium den without people feeling they are being *told what to do*?

Helpfully, I don't have an answer to this question so much as I have a commitment to making sure the conversation is had, that the question is being asked—over and over again, if necessary. How many decades did we need to grapple with cigarettes before "Four out of Five Doctors Prefer Camels" became "The Surgeon General Has Determined that Cigarette Smoking is Dangerous to Your Health"? And that conversation continues still.

For my family specifically, I hope many things. I hope my children have learned that you can do virtually anything you set your mind to, that big ideas are worth trying, and that your biggest support network is—ideally—your family. I hope they learned that healthy eating is a choice and that lots of things in life are bad for us—sugar, alcohol, reality television—but that often the key is awareness and moderation.

Lastly, I hope they learn that most things that are worthwhile—eating good food, raising happy children, having a fulfilling career—take time, thought, and energy. There are many shortcuts in life, but perhaps none that come free of consequences. Sugar is one of those things we have manipulated into giving us lots of shortcuts: to better taste, to more convenience, to ever-higher food industry profits. But at what costs? As the old saying goes, if you don't have your health, you don't have anything.

Me? For one thing I'm a better cook now. If pressed, I can make my own mayonnaise, kill a chicken, cook potatoes on an open hearth, and make desserts without fructose. Heck, I might even pour out the mac and cheese noodles a few seconds before the timer goes off, but I'm not promising anything. And I'm willing to try a lot more new things, although I've definitely crossed beaver off the list.

THE NEW NORMAL
— BY STEPHEN SCHAUB —

Throughout our Year of No Sugar, I say now without hesitation, my love and respect for my wife and her vision grew in new and amazing ways. Watching her explore and learn more about food, our society and its relationship to food, and the health consequences that result was inspiring. On several occasions, Eve visited our children's school and explained to their classes why we were doing this project and the science behind our decision. I am sure for our kids it provided an easy out when explaining why they could not have any sugar-added food: my mommy is crazy.

Now that the "official experiment" is over and several months have passed since it ended, I am happy to say that we have settled into what I feel is a positive "normal" for our family—somewhere in between A Year of No Sugar and where we started, before we watched Dr. Lustig's YouTube video. Eve still makes most meals from scratch, uses dextrose instead of sugar whenever possible, and we limit the number of desserts our family eats. I feel much more aware of what I eat, and I try to make positive choices for our family not based on a fear of food—or a fear that Eve would kill me—but rather science and common sense. More than anything else, what I've taken away from our Year of No Sugar is the realization that most people in our society don't really eat *food*. Not really. And I find it very sad that we as a society just stand by and watch each other poison ourselves day after day.

My father, of course, would have *loved* this project. In fact, I imagine it would have been very difficult to keep him at bay, as he would have flooded Eve and me with articles and ideas on a daily basis. His lifelong pursuit of the perfect diet always seemed to go to the extremes, because he was an extreme kind of guy. But what I have learned is that it is the food industry in our country that is really the extreme; eating local, fresh food—*not* loaded with needless added sugar, preservatives, additives, chemicals, and general crap—is really what should be considered normal. Because it *is* normal. It was normal for thousands of years. Perhaps this could have been a diet or lifestyle change my father could have lived with—I don't know. But I suspect he would be proud of us.

I've learned as much about myself and my family as I've learned about the crazy food system and myriad ingredients that are designed to make us give up. "Just eat it," we sigh all too often. "It isn't going to *kill* you." But to paraphrase Humphrey Bogart, no, sugar isn't going to kill you today or tomorrow, but someday it will, and for the rest of your life.

I've told a lot of stories in this book and I have just one more left to tell: when my girls were little—too young for school—they went one or two days per week for daycare to a lovely woman's house in a neighboring town. Locally, Martha's House is famous for being the kind of place everyone would want to go if they were a kid—her entire house is oriented toward children. There are bookshelves to the ceiling, armloads of puzzles, armies of Legos and Playmobil and Barbies. There is a record player with 45s, a piano, and several small outbuildings that are crammed top to bottom with old bicycles and enormous bins of clothes for dress-up. Every day the kids put on a play with the musical accompaniment of the record player such as "The Firebird," "The Three Little Pigs," or "Peter and the Wolf." There's an endless garden and an enormous sandbox and mini-trampoline, and a stream for shallow swimming, and apple trees that are perfect for climbing—I could go on and on. Heck, I figured, if *I* couldn't go to Martha's House, at least I could send my children there.

Martha herself turned seventy a year or two ago, but this slows her down not a whit—she has more energy than any grown adult I know and more than many children as well. She's been watching children at her house since her own four children were little a couple decades ago. Martha has seen it all. She's seen food fads come and go too—back in the seventies, she reminded me at one point, people were getting worried about too much sugar in their children's food. This worry was then successively supplanted by lots and lots of other worries—artificial colors and flavors, plastics, vaccinations, peanut allergies, gluten and dairy intolerances, and of course, high-fructose corn syrup.

Many moons ago, perhaps back when I was of an age when Martha could've changed *my* diaper, she got it into her head that, between home celebrations and school celebrations, children were getting an awful *lot* of sugar on their birthdays. In an effort not to compound the matter any further, she invented a Martha's House Specialty: Birthday Bread.

Nary a child's birthday goes by at Martha's House that is not marked by the preparation of these wonderful simple loaves. Each child helps with the mixing of the dough and is given a portion to knead and shape into whatever they wish: a bun, a little turtle, an initial. If a child has been absent during their birthday for some reason and returns, Martha always makes sure the child gets to make up their birthday bread. Not that the children would let her forget—they adore this tradition, just as they adore Martha, as they adore Martha's House and everything about it.

Are there any sprinkles on the birthday bread? Icing? Chocolate chips? Raisins at least? Nope. It's *bread*. Martha lights a candle in it at lunch and the kids sing "Happy Birthday," and as with everything at Martha's House, it's terribly festive. And God forbid a child's parents *forget* to bring that last leftover crumb home in their labeled paper bag to finish later—they will surely be forced by the wailing and lamentation from the backseat to return and claim the prized commodity.

Not that we can't have cake. Not that we can't celebrate. But we have to remember the lesson that Martha teaches in everything she does: kids *know* what's special. They know when you care. And it doesn't *always* have to involve sugar.

P.S.

W e're driving. It's January. Steve and I are driving through sloppy, foggy weather to have a date night—a movie at the theater in Glens Falls—when suddenly the perfect symmetry of it all hits me: Wasn't this exactly what we were doing at the beginning of the No-Sugar Project two years ago?

Now the book about our year is nearly done. Sort of. Are you ever really done with something that changes your life? As we drive, I compare our evening two years ago to tonight: *that* night we had been trying to see *True Grit* and failed because we could find no place to eat at fast enough to make the movie time. Tonight, we're on our way to see *The Silver Linings Playbook*, and we *will* make the movie: we ate dinner at home before leaving.

Back then we ended up having sausages at the German restaurant; tonight I had leftover spaghetti with sweet potatoes and ricotta; Steve had baked chicken with hot sauce because he's on another food rampage—attempting to lose spare pounds à la the Atkins diet. At the theater, I pass on the circus-y concession stand as usual, while Steve gets a "small" diet soda that is large enough to come with its own hand truck. I think, *The more things change, the more they stay the same.*

It makes me pause once again to reflect—so where *are* we now with all of this, now that it's been a full year since the project ended? What has truly stuck?

Speaking for myself, I am happy to no longer be the Sugar Nazi, or the Sugar-phobe; instead, I guess I can best characterize myself as a Sugar Avoider of the first order. I haven't lost my habit of obsessive label reading, haven't stopped counting how many items contain sugar on Ilsa's lunch tray at school or in the cart in front of me in the supermarket line. I haven't stopped being aghast. I still can't bring myself to buy things that I used to prior to our No-Sugar Year—shelf-stable tortillas, jar tomato sauce, dried cranberries, or the occasional pack of Fig Newmans.

But I have relaxed considerably. I don't have to make the agonizing choice to have nitrates instead of sugar in my bacon, or to buy the kids potato chips instead of whole-grain muffins. I can be reasonable and weigh one poison against another, choosing the lesser of all present evils. I still buy and use dextrose, but by the same token if a recipe calls for one tablespoon of sugar, I may very well put it in. Or not. Most of all, I find we avoid the mindless sugar consumption—the crappy store-bought sheet birthday cake, the supermarket cookies someone puts out at the board meeting, even homemade stuff I know I won't *really* love. We save actual sugar for the "worth it" stuff, stuff that is truly meaningful—for birthdays, at special occasions, that wonderful piece of chocolate after a meal. Who knows? Maybe a perfect, shining piece of Napoleon will one day come my way. If it does, I don't want to be sated with Cocoa Puffs and Snapple—I want to be *ready*.

Meanwhile, we've made our way into the theater, and we're seated in the ridiculously plush reclining theater seats and watch as the room darkens. The screen illuminates a scene intended to make us feel we are on a roller coaster: the virtual car the audience is in rides disembodied in space; it ascends into a star-filled night, dropping dramatically, and whips around corners to be abruptly confronted with Stonehenge-scale versions of items available at the concession stand: Giant Cokes! Living-Room-Size Boxes of Sour Patch Kids! Gargantuan Packages of Junior Mints!

Yep, I think. *Those folks on the roller coaster really* are *us.*

RECIPES FROM A
YEAR OF NO SUGAR

We would never have made it through our Year of No Sugar without a few key recipes that came to the rescue time and time again. Fortunately, I have an embarrassingly large cookbook collection, so when we were in need of, say, a no-sugar tomato sauce, I turned to my most dog-eared volumes for a recipe I could warp and mangle to meet our needs. Sometimes this was surprisingly easy. Other times it took a little bit more finagling. I offer this section not so much to claim any genius as a chef—(Yes!! I invented hummus! That was *me*!!)—but rather as one more piece that fills in the picture puzzle of our year.

A few months in, we were delighted to discover David Gillespie's subscription website howmuchsugar.com, which is filled with no-sugar recipes, most of which David credits his wife, Lizzie, with devising. I personally think Lizzie should have her own cookbook, reality cooking show, and James-Beard-themed bouncy house. Her recipes are reliable, delicious, and so well-crafted that no one I served them to ever suspected for a moment that they were enjoying a dessert that lacked sugar. Two of my favorites, Coconut Cake and No Sugar Shortbread, are reprinted here by permission.

Some recipes simply come from my bedraggled binder of ripped-out magazine pages, Internet tidbits, and handwritten family favorites. In these cases, I have altered directions here and there to reflect how *I* make them. I hope you will adjust them too, to find what works best in your house.

Even if you aren't going fructose free, every little bit we can get away from added sugar—every sandwich we can eat without sugar-containing mayonnaise, sugar-glazed cold cuts, and sugar-fortified bread—is some kind of progress. Every cookie we eat that *doesn't* contain granulated sugar, fruit juice, molasses, *or* honey, it all helps by putting just that much less toxin in our bodies. And who knows? We may even start to *like* it. You never know.

After-School Hummus

Kids love snacks, but snack time can be difficult on No Sugar: granola bars, vegetables with store-bought ranch dressing, fruited yogurts and juice are common "healthy" options that all get ruled out. To solve this, for after-school snacks, we alternated between big bowls of homemade hummus with vegetables, fresh fruit and cheese, and fresh-popped popcorn (sprinkled with olive oil or butter and nutritional yeast).

- → ¼ cup olive oil
- → 2 tablespoons fresh lemon juice
- → 2 tablespoons tahini (sesame seed paste)
- → 1 teaspoon ground cumin
- → ¾ teaspoon kosher salt
- → 1 15-ounce can chickpeas, rinsed
- → 2 cloves garlic

Puree all ingredients above in a food processor until smooth. Add between 1 and 2 tablespoons water and continue to puree until you reach a nice, creamy consistency. Put in a bowl for serving with vegetables or crackers. (Note: Crackers can be unexpectedly dangerous for the sugar abstaining, but we favored Triscuits—the original plain ones—which have no sugar and a wonderfully short list of ingredients as well.)

Optional: To up the "pretty" factor, drizzle with olive oil and/or sprinkle with a dash or two paprika. In my house, the bowl is usually licked clean before I get to this part.

My Favorite Tomato Sauce

Tomato sauce is a perfect example of a store-bought product that virtually *always* contains sugar, yet is very simple and cheaper to make at home without sugar *and* it will taste better to boot. This recipe makes about 4 cups of sauce, which can be used in everything from lasagna to soup.

→ 3 tablespoons olive oil
→ 4 garlic cloves, minced
→ 1 28-ounce can crushed tomatoes
→ 1 14.5-ounce can diced tomatoes

Cook oil and garlic in a medium saucepan over medium heat until it smells good, but before the garlic begins to brown. Stir in all the tomatoes with their juice. Let simmer until thickened, between 15 and 20 minutes.

Oil and Vinegar Salad Dressing

The main trick to avoiding sugar in your salad dressing is not to buy the premade stuff at the store. In Italy, I loved that they *always* had oil and vinegar, salt and pepper on the table—voilà! Salad dressing. Our friend Fabrizio once showed us the proper order for dressing one's salad: olive oil first, then salt and pepper, and finally drizzle the vinegar on top. There was a logic to it that I can't quite recall: Was it that the oil protected the lettuce leaves from the vinegar's acidity? That the vinegar dissolved the salt? Whatever the rationale, he was right—it always tastes best in this order.

In place of vinegar, a delicious alternative I used often at home is a healthy dose of fresh-squeezed lemon juice.

Oatmeal Sandwich Bread

Store-bought sandwich bread is another item that is nearly *impossible* to find without sugar. If you aren't lucky enough to have a *real* baker in your neighborhood—one who makes bread from ingredients you can count on one hand—this is an easy-to-make standby that I bake about once per week. I got this recipe, handwritten, from our friend Randy, the one who raises 52 chickens every year. (I substituted barley malt syrup for the originally called-for honey.)

→ 1 cup old-fashioned oats
→ 3 cups boiling water
→ 1½ tablespoons active dry yeast
→ 2 teaspoons kosher salt
→ 2 tablespoons olive oil
→ ½ cup barley malt syrup (available at health food stores)
→ 2 cups whole-wheat flour
→ 5 cups all-purpose flour

In bowl of mixer, put the cup of oats. Pour boiling water over oats and let sit one hour.

At one hour, sprinkle the yeast, salt, and olive oil on top. Add the barley malt syrup and mix with dough hook. Stir in whole-wheat flour. Stir in 2 cups of all-purpose flour. Then stir in 2 more cups of all-purpose flour, ½ cup at a time, mixing in between each addition.

Turn dough out onto a floured surface for kneading. Use final cup of flour to add to dough whenever it gets sticky. Knead for five full minutes, until dough has absorbed most of the final cup of flour and feels smooth. Place in a bowl and allow to rise for one hour.

Butter two loaf pans and heat oven to 350°F. After the hour has passed, turn dough onto counter, cut in half, and place each half in a bread pan. Allow to rise another 30 minutes.

Bake at 350°F for 33 minutes. Remove bread from oven and allow to sit five minutes before turning loaves out and letting cool on a rack.

Easy Homemade Mayonnaise

Another tough one: Mayonnaise. You just *can't* find No-Sugar Mayo at the store, but we certainly weren't prepared to go a whole year without it. I was intimidated. Wasn't homemade mayonnaise one of those things you had to be a real *chef* to make? Not so. If you have a Cuisinart, you will be amazed at how easy it is.

→ 1 egg
→ 1 teaspoon mustard
→ ½ teaspoon salt
→ ¼ teaspoon pepper
→ 1½ teaspoons white wine vinegar
→ 1 cup canola oil

Place all ingredients except oil in food processor. Process 15 seconds. With the motor running, add the oil in a consistent stream. (If you are using a Cuisinart, there is a hole in the white plastic plunger designed just for the purpose of funneling in oil at a nice steady pace so your mayo turns out perfect.)

Fresh, homemade mayonnaise lasts about three days.

Apricot Lemon Date Bars

My earliest experiments with No-Sugar Baking all involved dried apricots, dates, and bananas. This got old pretty quickly, with everything starting to taste the same. These bars, however, by far stood out as the best of the bunch. They're sweet, cakey, and great for hearty snacks or lunchboxes.

→ 2 cups chopped pitted dates and dried apricots
→ juice of 1 lemon
→ ½ cup water
→ ½ cup butter, softened
→ ¾ cup dextrose
→ 1 egg
→ 1 teaspoon salt
→ 1¾ all-purpose flour
→ ½ teaspoon baking soda
→ 1 cup rolled oats

Preheat oven to 350°F.

Place dates, apricots, lemon juice, and water in a saucepan. Cook on low heat—covered and stirring occasionally—for 10 minutes. Remove from heat and set aside.

In a bowl, cream together the butter and dextrose. Add egg and continue to mix. Stir in salt, flour, and baking soda. Finally, add the oats and mix with your hands. Press two-thirds of the crumbly dough into a greased 8- or 9-inch square baking pan. Spread fruit mixture over the dough. Take remaining dough and crumble over the top. Bake for 30 minutes. Cool in pan; cut into bars.

No-Sugar Poppy Seed Cake

This is my dad's all-time favorite cake, the one I made for his birthday in August—just slightly modified to use dextrose powder instead of sugar. (It goes very nicely with the cream cheese frosting in the following Coconut Cake recipe, but you'll want to make a double batch.)

- → ⅓ cup poppy seeds
- → ¾ cup milk
- → ¾ cup butter (1½ sticks)
- → 2 cups dextrose
- → 1½ teaspoons vanilla extract
- → 1¾ cups all-purpose flour
- → 4 tablespoons cornstarch
- → 2½ teaspoons baking powder
- → ¼ teaspoon salt
- → 4 stiff beaten egg whites

Soak poppy seeds in milk for one hour.

Heat oven to 375°F. Grease and flour two 8-inch cake pans. Cream butter then gradually add dextrose until fluffy. Add the milk and poppy seed combination. Add vanilla. Stir until evenly mixed. Sift dry ingredients together and then stir into the liquid ingredients. Mix until smooth. Carefully fold in the stiff beaten egg whites.

Pour batter into two cake pans equally. Bake in 375°F oven 20 to 25 minutes. Cool in pans 10 minutes and then remove.

Coconut Cake with Cream Cheese Icing

Vermont people love potlucks. LOVE them. And after discovering this cake, I took it to *every* potluck we were invited to. My idea was twofold: one, provide the only dessert my family could eat at the event (and head off any temptation otherwise) and two, take advantage of the anonymity of the potluck buffet to do some market research: *Would* anyone else eat it? *Could* it hold its ground against actual sugar desserts? Without fail, I returned home from each event with a *very* empty platter—not a crumb remained. Once, this cake went so fast that my kids didn't even *get* any and I had to promise I'd make another one when we got home!

Both the cake and icing come from David and Lizzie Gillespie's howmuchsugar.com.

- → 1 cup dried coconut
- → ¾ cup milk
- → 1 cup dextrose
- → 17½ tablespoons butter (2 sticks plus 1½ tablespoons)
- → 2 eggs
- → 1¾ cup all-purpose flour
- → 2 teaspoons baking powder
- → 1 teaspoon vanilla

Heat oven to 325°F. Soak the coconut in ½ cup of the milk for one hour.

Cream the butter and dextrose together until light and fluffy. Beat in the eggs, one at a time. Beat in the vanilla. Gradually add in the coconut mix.

Sift flour and baking powder together. Add half of the

flour to the butter mixture and mix only until combined. (It's important not to over-mix.) Add last ¼ cup of milk. Add last half of flour. Pour into a buttered, square baking pan.

Cook in the oven for 50 to 60 minutes. Let sit for 5 to 10 minutes before turning out onto cooling rack.

Cream Cheese Icing

→ 4 tablespoons (or 2 ounces) cream cheese
→ 2 tablespoons (or 1 ounce) butter
→ 1 cup dextrose

Beat cream cheese and butter until light and fluffy. Gradually beat in the dextrose until smooth. The consistency should remind you of peanut butter—if it is too thick, add a tablespoon or two of hot water. When cake is done cooling, frost cake on all sides.

No-Sugar Shortbread

Another treasured recipe from David and Lizzie Gillespie's howmuchsugar.com, and it's excellent for snack time and dessert time alike.

- → 1⅓ cup all-purpose flour
- → ¾ cup rice flour
- → 1 cup dextrose
- → ½ pound butter (room temperature)
- → pinch of salt

Heat oven to 300°F. Sift flour, rice flour, and dextrose together. Rub in the butter and then mix/knead into a smooth paste. Press into a single, flat layer, about ¼ inch in thickness, in a buttered casserole dish or rimmed cookie sheet. Prick with a fork in regular patterns.

Bake for 45 to 60 minutes, until coloring slightly. Remove from oven and cut while still warm. Shortbread will harden as it cools.

Heresy Pancakes

Pancakes are a BIG favorite in our house. We eat them pretty much every weekend, and if there are leftovers, I refrigerate them (or freeze them with a piece of wax or parchment paper between each one) so we can heat them in the toaster oven on a school morning during the week. Using banana and coconut is just one way of upping the sweetness, but you could try any number of different added-fruit combinations.

→ 2 cups all-purpose flour (or 1 cup all-purpose flour & 1 cup whole-wheat flour)
→ 2 tablespoons dextrose
→ 2 teaspoons baking powder
→ ½ teaspoon baking soda
→ 8 tablespoons powdered buttermilk
→ ½ teaspoon salt
→ 1 large egg
→ 3 tablespoons unsalted butter, melted & slightly cooled
→ 2 cups water
→ 2 very ripe mashed bananas
→ 4 tablespoons shredded unsweetened coconut
→ canola oil

Whisk together flour, dextrose, baking powder, baking soda, powdered buttermilk, and salt in a large bowl. In a separate bowl, whisk together egg, melted and cooled butter, and water. Add to these wet ingredients the mashed banana and shredded coconut. Whisk the egg and butter mixture into the dry ingredients until mixture is just incorporated. Don't overmix; a few lumps should remain.

Heat a skillet over medium heat and use small amount (1 tablespoon) of butter or canola oil to cook the cakes and add more as you go as needed. Use a ¼ cup measure to scoop batter onto hot skillet. Cook until bubbles begin to appear and then flip pancakes, cooking until they are nice and golden brown.

Dirt Cookies

We made a *lot* of cookies this year in an attempt to curtail our collective family sweet tooth. This recipe got the biggest raves of them all, from kids and grown-ups alike. Be sure to make them nice and big!

- → 1½ cups all-purpose flour
- → ½ teaspoon baking powder
- → ½ teaspoon salt
- → ¼ teaspoon nutmeg
- → 2¼ sticks unsalted butter, softened
- → 1½ cups dextrose
- → 3 large eggs
- → 3 cups rolled oats
- → 1 cup chopped dried apricots (unsweetened and unsulphured if you can find them)
- → 1½ cups raisins

Heat oven to 325°F. Whisk together in a small bowl the flour, baking powder, salt, and nutmeg.

In an electric mixer, beat together the butter and dextrose on medium speed until light and fluffy, about 4 to 5 minutes. Beat in the eggs one at a time until combined, about 30 seconds, scraping down sides as needed. Reduce mixer speed to low and slowly mix in flour mixture until combined. By hand, mix in oats, apricots, and raisins.

Working with ¼ cup dough at a time, roll dough into balls and lay on parchment-covered baking sheets (I use a Silpat), spacing them about 2½ inches apart. (I get about six cookies per cookie sheet.) Flatten cookie tops with your palm.

Bake until the tops of the cookies are lightly golden, but

the centers are still soft and puffy, 22 to 25 minutes, making sure to rotate and switch baking sheets halfway through. Let cookies cool on baking sheet for 10 minutes, then serve warm or transfer to a wire rack to let cool completely.

Fudge Brownies

This recipe was the Very Best No-Sugar Brownie after we tried several variations—we brought these to Greta's fifth grade class and they didn't leave a one uneaten. We enjoyed them most with carob chips until we realized carob was yet another processed sugar (whoops!). Anyway, they're great without chips too, and of course, you could always add some toasted nuts or maybe even raisins.

→ 1 cup (2 sticks) unsalted butter
→ 3½ cups dextrose
→ 4 large eggs
→ 1¼ cups cocoa (Dutch-process is best)
→ 1 teaspoon salt
→ 1 teaspoon baking powder
→ 1 tablespoon vanilla
→ 1½ cups all-purpose flour

Preheat oven to 350°F. Lightly grease a 9-by-13-inch pan.

Melt butter over low heat, then add dextrose and stir to combine. Crack four eggs into a bowl and beat them with the cocoa, salt, baking powder, and vanilla. Add the hot butter mixture and stir until smooth. Add the flour, and stir until smooth. Spoon batter into greased pan.

Bake for 35 to 40 minutes. Remove from oven and let pan cool on a rack before cutting and serving.

Birthday Bread

Once, in an effort to assuage some tears from one of my children who had missed a birthday-bread-making-Martha-Day, Martha gave me a copy of the recipe...and it is one of my treasured possessions. It's one of those wonderfully vague recipes that assumes you know how long to knead the dough by the feel of it and how to tell when your bread is done by the look of it. Like most bread recipes, it called for a few tablespoons of either sugar or honey, but I substituted dextrose here, which I have found works equally well in bread dough.

→ 1 package yeast
→ 2 cups warm water
→ 3 tablespoons dextrose
→ 2 teaspoons salt
→ ¼ cup oil
→ 7 cups flour

Add yeast and dextrose to the warm water and let stand 5 minutes. Add salt, oil, and flour a little at a time until you can work the dough with your hands. If sticky, add more flour. Knead.

Roll into ball shapes, letters, snakes, etc. To stick pieces together, brush with a little bit of water. Place on a cookie sheet and let rise 10 to 20 minutes. Bake at 350°F for 20 to 30 minutes, depending on the size of your shapes.

And for the Throwing-Caution-to-the-Wind crowd...

The Desert Island Desserts: What We Couldn't Live Without

A small number of our One Per Month Treat Desserts we enjoyed during our Year of No Sugar were *not* made by us at home. Others came from my favorite cookbooks, which I detail at the end of this section for those who are curious.

The three recipes listed below are the ones that are unique to me and our family—the kind you have tucked away on a stained index card in God Knows Whose handwriting and calling for weird things like hot water with baking soda dissolved into it. I treasure them, even as the called-for hunks of Crisco and mountains of powdered sugar now make me cringe. Nowadays I modify all my dessert recipes to include either no sugar or significantly less sugar, my favorite compromise being to substitute exactly *half* the sugar with dextrose. But here they are in their original form, as I made them on our monthly dessert days.

Great-Grandma Hotchkiss's Sour Milk Chocolate Cake with Buttercream Frosting
(January/April)
(aka Ilsa's-Turning-Six Chocolate Cupcakes/ Greta's Eleventh Birthday Cake)

→ ½ cup shortening (i.e., Crisco)
→ 1 teaspoon vanilla
→ 2 cups sugar
→ ½ cup cocoa
→ 2 eggs
→ ½ cup sour milk (½ cup whole milk to which you add ½ teaspoon white vinegar and dissolve in ¼ teaspoon baking soda)
→ 2 cups all-purpose flour
→ 1 teaspoon salt
→ 1 cup hot water with 1 teaspoon baking soda dissolved in

Heat oven to 350°F. Butter two 8-inch cake pans, cover bottoms with waxed paper cut to fit, butter and flour the wax paper.

In a mixer, cream shortening. Add vanilla, sugar a little at a time, cocoa, and eggs. Add sour milk and mix. Sift flour and salt together; add gradually to batter and mix. Lastly, add the hot water with baking soda, mix. Pour into two cake pans, dividing evenly.

Bake at 350°F for 30 to 35 minutes, until the cake begins to pull away from the sides of the pan. Cool on racks before removing from pans. Cool completely before icing.

Quick Butter Cream Frosting
(enough for one 8-inch two-layer cake)

→ 3 cups sifted confectioner's sugar
→ ¾ cup unsalted butter, softened
→ 4½ tablespoons milk
→ 1½ teaspoon vanilla

With a mixer on slow speed, combine all ingredients. Increase to moderate speed and beat until smooth. If frosting looks too thin, add more sugar to thicken.

Eve's Childhood Rhubarb Pie
(May)

Crust[67]:

- → 1⅓ cups all-purpose flour
- → 1 stick (8 tablespoons) unsalted butter
- → 1 teaspoon salt
- → 1 tablespoon sugar
- → ¼ cup ice water

Cut the stick of butter into 8 tablespoons. Put all the ingredients except ice water in work bowl of a Cuisinart. Process 5 to 10 seconds.

With machine running, pour ice water gradually through the feed tube in a slow stream. You may not need to use all the water. Watch the dough, and when it is the right consistency, it will form a ball. You will need two batches of this dough for the rhubarb pie: one for the shell and one for the top crust.

Pie:

- → 1½ cup sugar
- → ¼ cup all-purpose flour
- → ½ teaspoon nutmeg
- → 1 tablespoon butter
- → 2 eggs
- → 4 cups rhubarb, cut into 1-inch pieces

---

[67]This pie crust comes from a tattered scrap of paper in my recipe collection. It's the only pie crust I ever use—very easy, and I always get compliments on it. It works equally well with dextrose substituting for sugar.

Heat oven to 450°F. Roll one batch of the crust dough out, place in a 9-inch pie pan.

Sift together the sugar, flour, and nutmeg. With a fork or pastry blender, work in the tablespoon of butter as thoroughly as possible. In a separate bowl, beat the two eggs, then add to mixture.

In bottom of pie pan, place rhubarb on the crust, and pour egg mixture over the rhubarb. Cover with either a flat or lattice crust, remembering to add vents if using a flat top. Brush all pastry tops with milk or cream. Sprinkle all surfaces with sugar.

Bake at 450°F for 10 minutes. (At this point, I like to put a crust protector or a layer of tin foil over the top of the pie in order to prevent the highest parts of crust from getting overly done.) Reduce temperature to 350°F and bake 40 minutes more, or until pastry is browned.

Grandma Sharon's
Best-Ever Christmas Cookies
(December)

- → 1½ cups butter (3 sticks, softened)
- → 2 cups sugar
- → 4 eggs
- → 2 teaspoons vanilla
- → 5½ cups sifted, all-purpose flour
- → 2 teaspoons baking powder
- → ½ teaspoon salt

Heat oven to 375°F.

Cream butter and sugar together. Add eggs and vanilla; beat until light and fluffy. Sift together flour, baking powder, and salt, and stir into batter. Chill dough thoroughly.

Roll dough out 1/8 inch thick (the thickness is key!) and use cookie cutters to make shapes. Bake 8 to 10 minutes or until just *faintly* beginning to brown at the edges. Cool on racks. Decorate with icing or sprinkles as desired.

The recipes I got from cookbooks or elsewhere:

Chocolate Mousse (February) and **Pumpkin Pie with Whipped Cream** (November) came from *America's Test Kitchen Family Cookbook*.

Oh-My-God Sour Cherry Pie (March) came from *The Joy of Cooking* by Irma S. Rombauer, Marion Rombauer Becker, and Ethan Becker.

Emeril's Banana Cream Pie (September) came from *Emeril's New New Orleans Cooking* by Emeril Lagasse, but using the pastry cream from *Martha Stewart's Baking Handbook*.

Chocolate Peanut Butter Pie (October) came from www .evilchefmom.com.

ACKNOWLEDGMENTS

So one day, back in 2010, a very dangerous thing happened. I had this *idea*—which was the beginning of a long journey that ends with this page, more or less. First of all, I have to thank my daughters, Greta and Ilsa, who surprised, amazed, and inspired me, even while I quietly fretted I was ruining their lives. Now that a little time has passed, I have greater confidence that, in fact, our Year of No Sugar will be merely added to the list of "crazy things Mom made us do," which is likely to be very long, indeed.

I have to thank my friend Katrina Farrell, who I will always love for the fact that, when I told her about my idea of a No-Sugar Year, immediately volunteered to have her whole family do it right along with us. (Alas, being simultaneously gluten-free *and* sugar-free might just be harder than attempting to juggle feral cats. It was not to be.) She, along with her daughters, Stella and Lucy, spent a whole lot of our No-Sugar Year with us and gave us the gift of total acceptance.

Special thanks to my team of Super Friends who read this book's initial drafts and told me their honest-to-God-opinion-no-matter-what: Rhonda Schlangen, Robin Kadet, and Noreen Hennessy. You all steered me where I needed to go. How lucky am I to have you as friends?

I would be remiss not to thank the folks at school who helped me track down truly ancient data for the "school absences" chart: thank you so much to Mrs. Waterhouse and Mrs. Nelson.

I never would have made it through 2011 without the insight and support of David Gillespie, who has my deepest admiration for the work he has done promoting the facts and the message behind No Sugar. His book *Sweet Poison* appeared at an opportune moment in our year and gave me the desperately needed assurance that, in fact, I might just be the only one in the room who was *not* crazy. Also, his wife Lizzie deserves a Lifetime Achievement Award for that Coconut Cake alone.

My blog **Ayearofnosugar.com** formed the basis of much of this book, cataloguing our year as we went. I owe a great debt to the faithful readers and the frequent comment-posters whose stories and enthusiasm were deeply inspiring. Likewise thanks to bloggers David Gillespie (howmuchsugar.com), Betsy Shaw (numbmum.com), and Craig Goodwin (www .yearofplenty.org), who loaned me their enthusiasm when I desperately needed it, as well as so many of their wonderful readers by linking to my posts.

Of course, I must thank the man himself who started it all: Dr. Robert Lustig. Not only did he change our lives with that one daring lecture, but throughout our Year of No Sugar, he repeatedly astounded me by answering all of my inane email questions: every single one. I get the feeling that if Dr. Lustig thought he could solve the obesity epidemic by going from door to door and simply talking with people, one by one, he'd get out his comfortable shoes and start ringing doorbells.

Great thanks to Angela Miller, who, Clark Kent–like, changes from crack New York City literary agent to Vermont goat farmer in the blink of an eye: I don't know how you do it all, but I'm so very, very glad you do.

And deep gratitude to my editor Shana Drehs, who, with her red pencil wand in hand, is the fairy godmother of this book. Thank you for helping me find the carriage in the pumpkin patch.

Much love and appreciation to Mom and Dad. Dad, your Friday night pesto made me excited about food; Mom, your passion for words and getting them right made me excited about writing. So, basically, all of this is both of your faults.

Lastly I must thank my husband, Steve, who is my partner in everything, who reads what I write and always tells me what he thinks. Steve, the one-man tech team, without whom I could not tell the "up" end of a computer from a tin of anchovies. Steve, who could've looked at me that day, when I first proposed our "family project," and said just about anything but what he did say...

"A *whole year* without sugar? Hmmmmmm."

ABOUT THE AUTHOR

E ve O. Schaub lives with her family in Vermont and enjoys performing experiments on them so she can write about it. She was voted by her high school class "the funniest person Steve Martin has never met" and likes to spend her spare time wandering picturesque back roads composing limericks in Portuguese. She imagines it would be fun to win several important awards. She enjoys writing about herself in the third person.